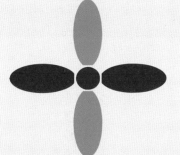

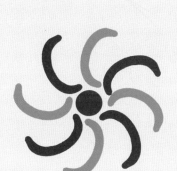

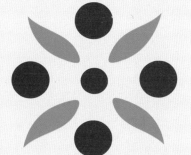

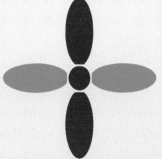

KUM NYE DANCING

Introducing the mind
to the treasures the body offers

Tarthang Tulku

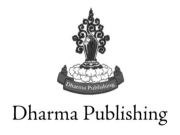

Dharma Publishing

Caution

Anyone who is pregnant, elderly, or has any kind of injury, health problems, or special conditions should not perform the heavier and more physical of these exercises. The dancing movements presented in this book should be studied only with the guidance of an experienced Kum Nye teacher.

Printed in the U.S.A. at Dharma Mangalam Press
Ratna Ling, California, 2012

Design/Layout: Raúl Bruno | Preciada Imagen, Inc. and Carolina Mazzocchi
Gestures performed by John Lozano
Photography by Jim McNulty

ISBN: 9780898000061
Library of Congress Control Number: 2012931585

The symbols used throughout this book are inspired by the symbols displayed on traditional thanka curtains, as well as on the clothes of lama dancers.

www.dharmapublishing.com   www.kumnyeyoga.com

Arnaud Maitland has been practicing and teaching Kum Nye for a long time, first with students at our Nyingma Institutes and now with participants in many other places around the world.

This book is dedicated to all of you and to all Westerners interested in spiritual practice.

CONTENTS

INTRODUCTION

When the energy of human embodiment is fully expressed,
it becomes art. It reveals our inner qualities, our distinctive flavors,
our souls. We become one with joy; the expression of joy
is our dancing.

I first introduced Kum Nye to Western students in the 1970s; during this period, at the Nyingma Institute, I gave the first Kum Nye exercises to a small group of professionals with backgrounds in psychology. I prepared this material in part as a response to questions these students had begun to ask about consciousness, awareness, meditation, and the senses. They wanted to understand many things that are not always addressed directly in Western thought: how the movements of the psyche relate to the movements and processes of the body; how consciousness experiences past, present and future; how karma operates; the nature of reincarnation; and the origins of things known in Western culture as psychic phenomena or miracles.

In contemplating their questions, I found no easy means to express my answers. Part of the problem was that I am not a native speaker of English, and my way of talking was sometimes hard for listeners to understand. But a deeper, more pervasive problem has to do with the English language itself. While English has developed a matchless vocabulary for the discussion of physical, mechanical, and business matters, it is not as well-equipped to translate the contents of many Buddhist texts, which contain a type of concepts that can be entirely alien to Western audiences. I felt that it would be necessary to simplify in order to communicate these concepts effectively.

As I worked with these first American and European students, it seemed to me that the Western mind needed more than a spiritual perspective, or tools for psychological and philosophical analysis, for the Westerners I encountered did not seem to know how to relate directly to their own bodies. This disconnection was making the basic practice of meditation and relaxation challenging. For this reason, I felt it was important to help students learn new approaches to the body and its responses to the world.

Working with the body, learning how to tune experience allows the mind to take a comfortable seat, creating space for the development of samatha and vipassana, calmness and clarity—keys to the emergence of transcendent awareness. Without this basic seat, it is difficult to cultivate the qualities that support a spiritual practice. When body and senses are in tune, our physical experiences can be friends and helpers, rather than obstacles to development. For this reason, yogic practice has from the beginning been regarded as a key prerequisite for more advanced Buddhist study.

In early times Buddhism had numerous powerful, even legendary yoga practitioners, and a deep and sophisticated yogic tradition handed down through texts as well as direct transmission. After Buddhism came from India, Tibet developed its own related yogic systems and terminology, producing an intricate map of the human body's subtle energy.

Tibet's esoteric Tantric texts contain rich and deeply considered instruction in how to follow the yogic path, how to use experience as a vehicle for realization. Yet at the same time, these texts offer little by way of systematic explanation or step-by-step guidance. They do not necessarily provide an accessible gateway to the training, especially for Westerners.

Kum Nye begins at a more basic level. It works with aspects of human experience sometimes known as the five skandhas; physical forms, sensations and feelings, perceptions, ideas, and sense of self are part of our ordinary experience, and fit comfortably within Western frameworks for understanding human being. Kum Nye's approach is congenial to this Western understanding, but at the same time it introduces new ways of thinking about and paying attention to embodiment. As it explores the layers of experience, it is able to provide simple but effective ways to work with special points, known in the yogic tradition as dharmachakras that are linked to the physical body and mediate many forms of energy. Kum Nye energizes the principal chakras, found in the belly, chest, throat, and head; at the same time, it engages many factors Westerners might find more familiar, including aspects of posture, breathing, the circulation of blood, and body temperature, and examines the way these factors function together as a whole.

Balancing the many sides of our human nature brings comfort, stabilizes meditation, and opens the door to a direct experience of non-duality. As body and mind are synchronized, senses offer more nourishment, complementing one another. The body relaxes, the mind finds peaceful accommodation, and we become more capable, more sensitive, and more effective in the world around us.

Without this well-developed inner calm, it becomes easier for us to oscillate between extremes of emotionality—we cannot find a point of balance. Our bodies become more vulnerable to stress and illness, and our sense-experiences can provide little support. No matter how sincerely we may wish to practice a spiritual discipline, we find our feelings are jarring and unsettled; uncomfortable ourselves, we may end up disturbing those around us.

This unbalanced system can develop strong biases; we can end up based largely in our heads, or ruled by powerful impulses and emotions. Many of us are in a state of habitual, perpetual conflict with ourselves, as the different facets of our embodiment engage in ongoing arguments. While these varied parts of us ultimately want the same thing—to be at peace, to be comfortable—each one has, so to speak, a different opinion about how to accomplish this aim. Basic needs like sleep or nutrition may be ignored in favor of sensual pleasures, or a desire for excitement may relegate our deeper feelings to the sidelines. This way of treating ourselves can have painful long-term ramifications.

Human beings as a rule long for peace, space, and happiness. We spend our lives seeking positive experiences, and we dream of joy and fulfillment. But the way that our bodies and minds interact does not produce this result. Out of balance, we are beset by problems. And in a world that is itself out of balance, the path to equilibrium may seem mysterious.

Western people have had relatively few opportunities to study their minds and bodies in a serious way. They have not had much experience with the sometimes strenuous training that can be found in a developed yogic tradition. A tough, ascetic approach might appeal to some, but it may not be the best way to begin. Kum Nye's path is gentler, quieter. Its goal is to foster a cooperative spirit between mind and body, by introducing mind to the riches the body offers.

Each sense has its own tone; each tone, a quality of its own. With practice, each quality becomes flexible, conducting us to greater and greater openness. Over time, as flexibility increases, we learn that we have the power to nourish ourselves at every moment. We find we need less and less outward support to provide sweetness to our senses and feelings; we do not have to rely upon pleasurable experiences in order to know joy.

In time, as we begin to touch greater depths in our practice, joy becomes part of us, an experience we can evoke at any time. The flexibility we have acquired through our training allows joy to express itself freely in our bodies and feelings, even during times of hardship. As this capacity for joy is developed and refined, even difficult experiences can be transformed. This need not take place through bodily channels or changes to our material circumstances; it can be done instantly, through emotions and sense-experience. Yogic practice enables us to distill the flavor of bodily experience into a potent form that can be brought directly to the present moment. In this way, even moments of deep calm or transcendent insight that we have known in other times can return, not as faint memories but as genuine internal events. If we reflect on this, we can catch a glimpse of a very different world, with a deeper flexibility to space and time than we may have imagined possible.

In our own way, we can follow the inspiring example of this advanced training. When we have hard times, we too can embody a joy that will sustain us through difficulty. This form of practice is not the same as escapism or a bullying attempt to feel good, no matter what. It depends upon flexibility, and it cultivates flexibility; through it, we become more, not less responsive to what is taking place. Gradually, we may come to regard hardship as an entirely positive opportunity, a challenge to refine our understanding and strengthen our ability to live peacefully, and to foster peace around us.

The first step is to learn how to get seated in experience. We can think of yogic development as a gradual settling down into this seat. At the beginning, we may only receive little tastes of this quality, but over time, as we continue to exercise, we encounter a calmness that does not disperse easily when thoughts or sensations come. It becomes possible to remain: to remain in calmness, to keep our seat. Our sense-experiences, our thoughts and feelings, come and go, but calmness is our steady companion, allowing us to make contact with the subtle, balanced, sustaining depths of practice.

Eventually, we learn to carry a much longer charge in the "battery cell": we become our own natural resource. We do not feel compelled to escape our circumstances, or find a refuge from the world. Instead of seeking help exclusively from teachers, therapists, or counselors, we can consult within our own experience, and counsel ourselves. When troubles come, we are able to adjust or even substitute the feeling-tones of our choice. By doing this, we fund the power to actively engage even unpleasant or unfamiliar experiences.

Over the years many of us have been trained, consciously or unconsciously, to react fearfully to new things. Confronted with the need to develop a new skill, live in a new place, or change a deep-seated habit, we may panic or close down emotionally. We may find ourselves unable to act for fear of making mistakes. As a result, many of us develop negative associations with unfamiliarity, for it always seems to bring agitation, suffering and confusion. But resilient and protected by our practice, we are well-equipped to deal with a broader range of situations, even unfamiliar ones. When we are faced with the new, we can respond creatively. Reaching into our own depths, we can combine ingredients to produce a beautiful experience. The flavor of what is happening changes. The clarity and joyfulness we create show us our situation in a new light, and agitation subsides. It is not necessary to go hunting around for healing: we possess healing qualities within ourselves. Kum Nye can help us to discover them, and practice can help them to emerge and become active in our lives.

Kum Nye teaches us how to use all our senses, all our thoughts, and all facets of our experience. Working in this way, we can produce not only more beneficial physical sensations, but better, more balanced intellectual concepts, deeper awareness, and healing for the mind, as we cultivate calmness and clarity. All of these benefits are potentially available; but first, we start with the body. The body offers us powerful ways to quiet the mind; the soothing qualities we discover in our bodily experience have the power to influence our thinking, where our instructions and admonitions may have no effect.

As we practice, we may end up telling ourselves, "I'm not doing this right." "I don't know how to do it." "If I go on, I might lose myself." "I'm confused." "I don't know what it means to relax." These anxious thoughts might seem deep and probing, yet they are actually ways to continue to hold onto our self-orientation.

There is another way; we can more openly experience the varied flavors of our sense of feeling. Instead of accepting some parts and rejecting others, instead of hanging on to our assumptions about ourselves, we can get in touch with our most neglected sides, gently massaging them, opening up these parts of our bodies and minds and receiving the gifts within them. We may be very different, at heart, than we imagined.

As Kum Nye communicates a different aura to our experience, our deeply-held sense of identity begins to change at its core. As our thought processes slough off their characteristic anxiety, becoming more neutral, thinking no longer poses an obstacle to being. The nucleus of the self opens up, and treasures emerge. Ego identity, self-image, worry, guilt—practice can gradually soften the intensity of our attachments, introducing new flavors. If the bonds to our orientations could be loosened up, we would receive a huge bonus. Enormous quantities of energy would be set free, and our awareness, instead of being tethered to subjects and objects, could expand more and more widely. There are many positive qualities locked inside our ego—depths of feeling, talent and intelligence. Free of fear, released from the constraints of our subjective orientation, we can express these qualities in new ways.

We can cultivate and protect our inner resources, so they never run dry. When they are fully developed, we won't have to hang on to hope, put our faith in a misty ideal, or dogmatically convince ourselves that our path is the correct one. We can have total confidence, based on the evidence of our senses. The best route to this more open way of life is the practice of stillness. But even in sitting practice, we do not "hold still." Stillness comes as a result of loosening up long-standing tension; like a ball that slowly rolls to a stop, we slowly smooth out, and the oscillations of our senses and emotions, bit by bit, subside. At first, sitting may be somewhat unfamiliar; certain exercises and practices can help to stabilize the sitting posture and make it more comfortable. As we sit, we bring in many nourishing feelings, adjusting and harmonizing our posture. When our sitting grows more settled, and calmness and quietness have taken root, then it is possible to dance.

As we engage the flow of feeling, each technique, gesture, and posture becomes a form of creative expression. The movements of our bodies begin to communicate deep experiences of wholeness; our gestures manifest the alignment of body and mind. When the energy of human embodiment is fully expressed, it becomes art. It reveals our inner qualities, our distinctive flavors, our souls. We become one with joy; the expression of joy is our dancing.

Discovering Kum Nye dancing

The exercises in this book are new. I first started to develop them in 2008 to help my students remain relaxed and flexible for long periods of hard physical work outside. These original exercises were refined in mid-2009, as this small, dedicated group of volunteers undertook a massive book production project. For twelve hours a day or more, they collated, wrapped and boxed thousands of sacred texts to be offered to ceremony participants at Bodh Gaya, India. This is strenuous work; the hands and wrists are taxed, legs and feet become sore, and heavy lifting takes its toll on the back. The work, performed largely in silence in an extremely disciplined temple environment, was also mentally challenging, requiring patience, commitment, and precision. At the height of their activity, these volunteers were wrapping six thousand books a day; to accomplish their goals, they had to summon deep reserves of energy and enthusiasm.

I practiced outdoors with these students every afternoon, leading them in special exercises. These exercises gave people a break from the repetitive movements and postures of collating, wrapping and boxing; they also allowed people to enjoy some fresh air and shake out their fatigue. Every day, I introduced another exercise. As people practiced, they found they liked the movements and became interested in learning more about them. Eventually, my student John Lozano, who has taught dance for many years, worked with Arnaud Maitland to develop the movements into connected groups.

These were not precisely traditional Kum Nye postures, but instead were based on temple practices I had known as a young man in Tibet; as I worked, I drew upon my recollections of exercises that were used to prepare for the sacred ritual movement colloquially known as lama dancing.

Traditional lama dancing uses physical choreography to open up the self and liberate energy for Dharma activity; these exercises, intensifying feeling in similar ways, can tame our resistance, resentment, and lack of cooperation. The postures and practices in this book, therefore, are not exactly massage. They are invigorating rather than soothing, designed to energize the body and to wake up consciousness. This kind of coordination produces greater cooperation—both with other people, and with ourselves.

As human beings, we come to know the world through many filters and structures, ranging from the shapes of our sense organs to the cultures in which we are raised. Our responses to the world around us, once fresh and spontaneous, gradually get stuck in channels of habit, hardened into place by years of repetition. Our personalities, too, begin to harden, as we allow ourselves to be governed by these habits and the likes and dislikes they have helped to put in place.

Yogic practice has the potential to alter greatly this channelized character of experience; exercising the body strongly in this way opens up sometimes startling alternatives to our ordinary approaches to life. It generates an effect that is immediately tangible at the feeling and energy level. By intensifying bodily experience through movement and posture, it is possible to address impacted parts of ourselves directly and decisively.

Earlier presentations of Kum Nye have tended to be slow and introspective. They are well-suited to quiet, solitary practice and were designed to be done easily in the bedroom or private study. The practices presented in this book, in contrast, point outwards; dynamic, dramatic, even occasionally a little silly, they emphasize the transformative power of yoga, and present an opportunity to make real and meaningful changes in our energy levels, our patience and tolerance, and our physical and mental flexibility.

Chapter One

Our human set-up

Kum Nye is more than an exercise regime; it is a system of embodied knowledge. If it is practiced deeply and sincerely, it can lead to a transformation of the human condition.

Opening the gate

In the West, most people associate the term "yoga" with a set of prescribed movements or postures which are supposed to reduce stress and improve health and well-being. But yoga is more than an exercise regime; it is a system of embodied knowledge. If it is practiced deeply and sincerely, it can lead to a transformation of the human condition.

The origins of classical yoga as a spiritual practice go back at least as far as the second century BCE in India, when Patanjali, the founder of Raja Yoga, authored the Yoga Sutras. Hatha Yoga, founded in the fifteenth century, developed the now-familiar concept of asanas, or discrete body postures. Hindu forms of yoga first came to the West in the mid-nineteenth century, where they gradually gained in currency, finally entering mainstream culture in the mid 1960s. Since then, yoga in the West has evolved into a largely non-religious body-mind discipline with practitioners of all ages.

In recent years, Tibetan forms of yoga have become more familiar to Western audiences. Tibet has a long and vibrant tradition of yogic practice that is deeply integrated with advanced spiritual practice; for over a thousand years, Tibetan masters of many lineages transmitted knowledge beyond concepts using the vehicle of human embodiment. Kum Nye is part of this lineage.

Kum Nye was designed to be gentle enough for first-time students and accessible to people of all ages, dispositions, and physical conditions. But although it is accessible, it is nevertheless an authentic yogic practice with deep roots. Kum Nye is often translated as "body massage." But Kum (sKu) means more than the physical body; it means substance, matter, manifestation. Nye (mNye) can mean "massage," but it also means wise usage, the action of tending and tuning. Nye (mNye) brings out the best in Kum (sKu), allowing it to develop into beauty.

Manifested through the senses

The texture of human experience manifests through the senses. Whether we are working, studying, taking care of our families, or relaxing, our bodies are part of every experience, every interaction we have. Experiences of comfort, of being sick, of pleasure or pain, all are mediated by our senses. A body may be alive, but without eyes, without ears, without the power of smell or taste, and without skin to sense, its experience would be desert-like; it would be hard to call such a mode of existing "life."

The body's five principal senses constitute our vehicle—our way of being alive. They connect us to the physical world, allowing us to find our way in space and time; they receive the world outside us on our behalf. Like party hosts, our eyes, ears, noses, tongues and skin bring guests into the home of the body, introducing us to visual forms, sounds, smells, textures, and tastes; these are crucial ingredients of our memories, thoughts, and feelings. A pleasant party atmosphere comes from the positive interactions of the hosts and the guests. When relations are good, we have good parties; in experience, it is the same. When our minds and bodies coordinate, we are comfortable, healthy, and happy.

How, then, do we harmonize and improve these relationships? Our traditional ideas tend to group experience into good and bad categories: good events produce good sensations, whereas bad events bring bad feelings. There is a predominant belief that illness, accidents, and hardship are going to give us unhappiness; there is nothing we can do about it but endure. This way of thinking is common in the modern world; and yet it is relatively easy to recall people we have known in fortunate circumstances who nevertheless seem very unhappy. And while it may be a little rarer, we may also know people who seem content even when their circumstances are hard. Some internal process must be taking place, some alchemy of experience that allows us to take profit even from hardship.

We know from experience that our bodies can be tuned. By changing our diet and adding some exercise, we can improve our energy, endurance, and flexibility. It is possible to tune our experiences in a similar way. Yogic practice offers us a wide range of ways to massage our experience, altering our relationship to the circumstances that impact our lives. The thought that we can subtly transform the quality of our ordinary experience encourages us to take a closer look at the interior structure of thoughts, feelings, and sensations; they may be far more complex assemblages than they might seem.

The mind-body interplay

For all beings, the senses are mediating experience. Our senses are the part of us that connects with the rest of the world, and each sense has its own specific, characteristic way of engaging and relaying its signals. The senses condition not just how we perceive, but also how we feel and think. While we share certain basic operations and structures in common, each sense faculty is distinct: no two people see the same thing in precisely the same way. Our age, health, and circumstances of physical embodiment affect our senses; but sense-experiences can also be profoundly affected by intangible factors. For example, odors, which might seem resolutely biological, are packed with personal and cultural associations. Different cultures celebrate different flavors and smells; our individual histories are also contributors, giving us powerful responses connected to where we grew up and what we experienced. The odor of burning charcoal might evoke in the mind a family outing, a fire danger, or a religious ritual, depending on our cultural background. We respond to these associations; we receive the same odor in different ways.

The interplay between mind and body is far from simple; the human set-up has many layers that work together to produce even our most basic and mundane experiences. The physical level includes the interplay of matter, energy, and space; the distinctive characteristics of our sense faculties, which take in certain signals and filter out or miss others; the operations of our internal organs; and the function of the breath. At the perceptual level, the set-up presents us with distinguishable objects: we see figures against grounds, and our senses point things out in space. The perception of time as directional gives rise to our deeply ingrained framework of cause and effect. At the cognitive level, human being is profoundly affected by the structures of language. We can also trace the effects of culture, upbringing, and past events as they shape each unique human experience. Finally, at the subtle energy level, the body is permeated by flows of energy that intersect at many different points.

While we can distinguish many different levels or aspects to the human set-up, they are in reality profoundly interconnected. It is for this reason that yogic practice, which can activate all the layers at once, can make deep and enduring changes in our experience through techniques of meditation, visualization, contemplation, movement, and breathing.

Those of us with some science in our background may be used to thinking about body structure, but the yogic traditions can also teach us to identify subtler structures—the structure of our sense-perceptions, the structure of our thoughts and feelings. In yogic practice, this complexity of our experience, the subtle interactivity of body and mind, is opened up and explored.

Yoga as union

Yoga is a Sanskrit word that originally meant "union" or "yoking." Yoga can be understood as a practice of unification: yoga yokes together the body, sensory perceptions, feeling, and mind. In traditional Eastern disciplines, yogic exercises are very important preliminary practices that lay the foundation for spiritual transformation; the seriousness with which they are treated reminds us that although yoga in the West has thus far mainly been aimed at improving physical health and calming the emotions, the potential exists for a far deeper engagement. Through yogic techniques of movement, meditation, visualization, and breathing, practitioners can touch subtle energy. Working at this level, the yogis of ancient times were able to refine and develop their psychic and spiritual energy, tracing the most delicate connections of body and mind.

Here in the West, we are not yet at that level; for the most part, we are only just becoming acquainted with these potentials. Kum Nye was developed to introduce a new relationship of mind and body; it uses ordinary, straightforward postures and begins by fostering harmony and positive feeling within the body. The exercises of Kum Nye reconnect us with our senses and help us wake up to the way our experiences take place; the exercises give us methods to relate more intimately with the world around us.

Connecting mind to the present

According to the yogic tradition, a healthy mind is one that knows how to inhabit the present moment. Undisturbed by memories of the past, free of fears in the present, and unconcerned with projections of the future, a healthy mind engages experience freshly and directly. Western psychological and therapeutic thought has come to respect the importance of the present moment for mental health; it is a common idea nowadays that the answer to many of our emotional problems is to "get present," to live in the moment. The present moment is the moment of embodiment. This is when the event takes place: this is the right now of our experience. We may assume that the present is where we live—yet are we present in the present? Are we truly living in the present tense? Instead of engaging the moment, we often seem to be engaged in reflections of reflections, as if we lived in a recursive mirror-maze, its passages turning endlessly in upon themselves.

The whirl of our ordinary thought processes—our plans, daydreams, and internal monologues—effectively assures that our awareness remains disassociated from the present moment. We are just too busy to be present. We are preoccupied, thinking something about something else; then we are busy thinking something about our reflections about that thought-of-something, inspiring further reflections and analysis until no thing is left—just wheels within wheels, and meanings of meanings. Fantasy, story, memory, plan, and concept: a great many of us live our lives moving from meaning to meaning, nomads in a wasteland of mental images. Reflecting upon reflections, we slip away from what is in front of our noses into comparisons, histories, and judgments. Yet many of us also have a feeling that our lives are being eaten up by worries and regrets—that we are living trapped in the past, or stuck in yearning for a future that never arrives. We understand instinctively that the only real nourishment available to us is in the present moment, yet we feel that we have been barred from access.

A curious effect of asking the question of what is actually happening when we are not present is that we begin to examine our experience openly and honestly. As we recognize that we are not present, the moment of recognition has the power to engage us in the now. It presents the present.

Chapter Two

Beyond instructions

If we are willing to relinquish control, to merge with our experience, we can touch a new openness. By letting go of our demands for certain results, we can gradually leave the corral we have created for ourselves. Opening up to ourselves, we enter a new adventure.

On orders to relax

How can we access the nourishment available in the present moment? We sense that relaxation is the key. Relaxation is a state of being we could call dynamic rest. Calm and flowing, peaceful yet alert, true relaxation expresses itself both in movement and in stillness. We see it clearly and profoundly expressed in the joyful behavior of animals; a cantering horse communicates its relaxation in fluid motion. When we are relaxed, we too are free to move. We do not brace ourselves against what we are experiencing, but are fully engaged within it. We know that relaxation could help us to feel better, to perceive more clearly, to live in alignment with ourselves and the moment of our experience. So we apply our analytical minds to the situation. Disconnection is identified as the problem; relaxation—getting into the present moment—is identified as the solution. And so we start to give ourselves instructions. We pepper ourselves with encouragements, corrections, scolding, imperatives—"I have to try to relax"—even direct commands, ordering ourselves to settle down, to stop being tense. Perhaps as a result of our efforts we quiet down for a time, yet there remains a subdued, almost subliminal tension. A dog that has stopped barking but is ready to bark at any moment may be quiet, but it is not really at rest or relaxed.

We have an image of what relaxation is like, something we can point to when someone asks us what the word means. We have an idea of what it means to be relaxed. Yet this idea is not itself relaxed in feeling, but quite fixed in character. If we look closely, we might be surprised to find that our notions of relaxation are pre-fabricated, sharply defined, closed up like boxes and frozen in place like poses. We know we need to relax; we tell ourselves so. But this recognition of the need to relax has a paradoxical quality; it may be keeping us separate from true relaxation, the union of mind and body that we seek.

Controlling mind

If we take a closer look at our experience of what is ordinarily called mindfulness, we may find an undercurrent of tense watchfulness. All too quickly, "being aware" becomes wariness. Our wariness, in essence, is awareness of something. We focus on an object that is scissored out by our perceptions and given great importance. If we look closely, this object of our attention seems to boil down to something we need, or something that might cause trouble. Deep inside, where the more ancient strata of our human being remain in operation, perhaps we are still feeling the desperate need to avoid danger and obtain the things that will enable us to survive. As a result, we can take a dictatorial attitude toward our experience, intimidating our own senses, pushing and pulling ourselves around in search of a desired state. Like a rough trainer trying to master an unruly horse, we put sensing in a corral called "relaxation." We insist that sensing stay in there, holding the pose that will make it better.

In this light, meditation, visualization, breathing, and the movements of disciplines like Kum Nye can come to be regarded as strategies to control our experience. Under the influence of controlling mind, healthy means "correct." Exercises can be done well only if they are correctly executed, following the rules. We can see this attitude widely reflected in conventional student and teacher roles, where instructions are issued, repeated, and obeyed. But this control runs deep within us, deeper than the cultural structures in which we are trained how to behave. For just as the trainer controls the horse, "I" controls "me." In our most basic operations as selves, we seek to control not only our thoughts, but our present sense of being.

This legacy of control may color our experience with Kum Nye at the beginning. Yet we can view the techniques of Kum Nye quite differently. For although they can be misinterpreted, turned by our controlling minds into a rigid system of instruction, at bottom they are tools, pointers to direct our attention, ways to engage. Kum Nye presents to us the textures of our physical sensations, and teaches us to pay attention to the quality of our breathing—through its exercises; these facets of our experience are brought vividly to present awareness. With training, we can pay attention in a more detailed way, carefully noticing the distinguishing marks of our experience, and tracing how they arise inside us.

Regimes of sensation

Kum Nye offers numerous methods for discovering how our experiences emerge. It teaches us to work in a subtle, gradual way with sensation and perception. When we begin to look at our feelings and sensations up close, our view might be hazy; we may not be able to see the developments and changes clearly. Gradually, however, practice refines our awareness, and we become more sensitive. While at first we may not have noticed, we come to realize that our sense-impressions are like living beings—they have lives and trajectories of their own. Our sensations have a quality of movement, rhythm, evolution. Over time, from faintest beginnings, perceptions take shape.

A sound comes; depending on our relationship to that sound, we might hear words, music, or a distracting noise. These connotations arise as the sound is received, absorbed, and processed by ears, nervous system, mind and memory. The images we see may be forming in a similar way; as connections to other images held within conscious and unconscious memory are sparked, as patterns are recognized, what we see slowly accumulates depth and significance. Our sensations, our thoughts, our feelings, associations, impressions and memories are guided into being through innumerable repetitions, assuming their characters according to a pre-existing pattern, within which each noise, each odor, and each flicker of light we see finds a home. As patterned productions, our experiences take their shapes and forms according to a regime of restrictions and conditions. Each experience derives its significance from a regime. These inner structures operate not unlike

∴

political parties, prescribing behavior and insuring that each member carries out the party's agenda. Insofar as each sensation has its own identifiable qualities and characters, it has been defined within a regime. It owes allegiance to its party—and our senses go along, aiding and abetting the operations of the regime.

All civilizations and cultures have styles of their own, approaches to living that are carried out, expressed in various ways by human beings. Our senses carry on these lineages, operating within the confines prescribed by each society, each subculture, each family, and each entwined moment of our individual past history. Each of us responds uniquely—yet these responses are nevertheless taking place through a form of regimentation, pattern-matching with the past. Established truths—"I dislike this kind of experience"—govern our perceptions, framing what takes place inside us. Without thinking about it too much, we might decide it's simply how things are with us. Yet all of these preferences, these ways of being, emerge from the regimes of sense; they have a lineage that can be traced. While we may feel very much at home within our likes and dislikes, our history and personality, we can also be trapped in subtle and frustrating ways. Objects appearing to the eyes are pre-defined, appearing within a pre-scripted position in the regimes of sense; sounds heard are promptly identified and given a context, filled with positive or negative connotations. Language shapes the thoughts that take place within it; feelings create their own consequences, and our well-being goes up and down, round and round, as a result. Westerners call this psychology; Easterners regard it as the operation of karma and klesa, deeply ingrained ways of being that reiterate and reproduce themselves, creating blockages that can last for lifetimes. Yogic practice, as it illuminates the operation of our sensations, feelings, and thinking, reveals the powerful influences coloring our experience, and transforms our sense of what is anchoring the reality of our perceptions, feelings, and ideas.

Understanding the roots

Instead of just looking at isolated experiences or events, accomplished yoga practitioners have learned to look at the way experience is being assembled.

Beneath the individual expressions of the sensations, they perceive the larger structures that frame what we see and how we see it. Yogis understand the intricate relationships between our senses and the world that exists beyond our skin; they can see how perceptions are formed, and how they operate as expressions of a pre-existing regime, connecting to past history, memory, feeling, conceptual awareness, and consciousness itself. In this way, the great yogis penetrated the roots of experience. Perceiving the sources of blockage, they could discern the correct antidotes. Identifying the branching of cause and effect, they could see the consequences of actions in advance.

Yoga practice is designed to illuminate these linkages, massaging them and bringing new relationships and hidden treasures to light. Working in subtle ways with the body can release blockages in the mind, bringing to light habits of manipulation, edifices of ignorance, and the turning wheels of our resentments. By working gently and precisely with the body, yogic practices can clean out and release these blockages. This attuning to and opening up subtle layers of presence is the essence of Kum Nye practice, as awareness merges with and illuminates our experience.

If we are willing to relinquish control, to merge with our experience, we can touch a new openness, waiting for us beyond words and concepts, beyond the framework of our habits. By letting go of our demands for certain results, relaxing our wariness, we can gradually leave the corral we have created for ourselves. Opening up to ourselves, we enter a new adventure, beyond the familiar and restrictive sensory experiences of "sweet" and "sour," beyond the known characters of our own habitual thinking.

Without instructions

Beyond the pre-patterned character of our experience, beyond instructions, there may exist a completely different reality—an entirely open field. Our conceptually oriented minds, operating in the ordinary, language-based way, pursue the goal of "relaxation." Yet that word finds no referent in the open field. There, all is already open; fixed concepts like "tension" and "relaxation" may not apply. It may seem, to

∴

our conscious minds, to be a distant ideal, and yet we can embody this perfect peace for ourselves; it is not an abstraction but a felt reality. Once we enter that openness, swimming in the blue, bottomless ocean, we are enfolded, naturally accommodated by our experience. Joining the flow, we become one with what we sense, emerging free from fear and desire. As we release our need to give ourselves dictation, we begin to sense a new possibility. It may be that in its essence, beneath its comparing and conceptualizing, the substance of the mind is open and flexible— part of the field of being. It is as if we said to space, "Hey, open up!" And space replies, "Me? I don't need to open up. I'm already open. Maybe you need to open up your perspective." We discover that we have what we need; we are what we seek. Like space, we are already open.

CHAPTER THREE

KUM NYE AS SENSORY CREATIVITY

Kum Nye practice becomes an opportunity to develop a deep knowledge of our individual embodiment, the specific expression of sacred energy called "myself."

Open fields

Knowledge of something tends to lock it up in a cognitive box; such knowledge, caught in subjects and objects, does not necessarily conduct us to openness. But yogic disciplines like Kum Nye foster awareness as union with what is perceived, felt, and known. This kind of knowledge can conduct us to openness. We begin to touch an unbounded continuum, one that reaches beyond the limited structures imposed by our concepts. This openness lies beyond our discriminating judgments, our pros and cons, our assessments of right and wrong; it lies beyond our concepts of "sensation," our narratives and ideas about experience—even beyond the subtle "nesses" that anchor the objects of our thinking.

As the body gains flexibility, as tissues soften up, so also do our senses, thoughts, and feelings; the hard casings of our habits begin to melt. Gradually, even the practitioner, the "I" directing, observing, yet separate from what is being sensed, begins to loosen up. In this way, Kum Nye can have a powerful impact on our being human. We can allow this freedom of movement to ourselves, to our experience of being "I." Obstacles and blockages that seem carved in stone, just the way things have to be, begin to disclose their developmental paths, in the process losing their hardness. The more closely we look at these phenomena, the more apparent it becomes that all these seemingly permanent structures—even the "I" itself—are expressions of energy.

Becoming bliss

The natural world offers us a powerful illustration of the fundamental malleability of our sense-experience. Water has the potential to assume many forms. Manifesting as ice, it can be wafer-thin and brittle, or miles thick and virtually permanent. Appearing as snow, it can be delicate and crystalline, slushy, or powdery. In clouds, in rain, in the ocean wave, in the subterranean stream—on our planet, water reveals an astonishing range of different characters. We can distinguish them because they differ in shape and form, yet we know that fundamentally they are all expressions of the substance known chemically as H_2O.

It may be that our experiences—the manifold textures and qualities that shape our lives—are not unlike the many manifestations of water. Thoughts, sensations, and emotional states could all be understood as expressions of a basic, fundamental openness. Like ripples and waves, some are strong and dramatic, some soft and subtle. As we practice, we learn how to expand the feelings stimulated by our exercise. We begin to see that all the shapes and forms we take as real parts of our experience—the feelings and sensations, the ideas and plans, and the dictating part of our minds—may be only surface phenomena after all. We can sense the ripples forming, spreading, traveling, and gradually dispersing, smoothing away into calmness. Penetrating the nature of experience, we enter an open field of awareness. This field is a space of manifestation; it is flat, like a field, not because it is abstract or dimensionless, but because it is free of hierarchies, histories, and structures. The open field expands beyond all limitation.

Kum Nye lets us touch that field of being. Kum (sKu) is body, a nexus of sensitivity; Nye (mNye) is a method of exercise that brings results—through Nye, the body experience is transmuted. The result of Nye is a floating quality sometimes called bliss—but this experience in truth has no name. It cannot be confined by the framework or structure of language.

Once we taste it, we no longer mistake the ersatz for the real experience. Knowing is union; we become one with our experience. It is no longer something to have or to lose. Becoming bliss is knowledge we can taste.

The Kum Nye laboratory

We can envision the practice of Kum Nye as the process of conducting experiments in a laboratory: close observation reveals different experiential feedbacks. Thinking of our practice as a form of knowledge-gathering through experimentation reminds us to approach Kum Nye with a spirit of open inquiry. There are no foregone conclusions here; we are creating knowledge we did not have before. Practicing alertly, we test each ripple, each expression of the field. Our bodies are active partners; they are not just the objects of our study but form the laboratory itself.

It is important to develop our own knowledge of our own bodies, for each body has a unique chemical structure, and its own distinctive ways to eat, sleep, and relate. Each body has different needs, different habits, and different ways to express itself. What helps one body to thrive may have an adverse effect on another body; working closely with ourselves, we can find the approach that is best for us. Our practice becomes an opportunity to develop a deep knowledge of our individual embodiment, the specific expression of sacred energy called "myself."

This empirical spirit can enrich our approach, encouraging us to pay close attention to how we respond to different practices, different exercises. If we embrace the spirit of laboratory study, we can experience the wonder of really getting to know ourselves, not as objects studied under a microscope, but inside out. We receive the gift of a lived awareness, and knowing becomes a form of intimacy with all we experience.

As we delve more deeply into these explorations, we learn that all experiences are expressions of fundamental unity. The gamut of physical shapes and forms, the subtle tissues of our emotional states, are all manifesting energy; they are active moments of creativity. As we trace the development of these myriad expressions, our sense of our role in the process begins to change. Is it possible that we could be creators of our own experience? Could we learn to manifest beauty and happiness, instead of waiting for it to be delivered to us by circumstance?

Sensory creativity

The great yogis of history did not need to seek pleasures or entertainments. Outwardly, they had few friends, and few possessions or comforts; some of them had nothing but a worn-out robe and a pot for boiling water. To their lay contemporaries, these yogis must have seemed to live lonely, solitary lives. Yet they were constantly entertained, enjoying every drop of their living experience. Even though they dwelled in austere, even harsh places—a little hut in the mountains, a practice cave—nevertheless, they were highly developed internally; they rejoiced in the sounds they heard, the flavors they tasted, the odors they smelled, the textures they touched, and the light they perceived.

These great practitioners knew how to foster a positive relationship between the outside world and their senses. Open and pure, embracing their surroundings without judgment, they found deep beauty and contentment even in difficult circumstances. Although we are only ordinary people, not realized yogis, we, too, can engage experience in transformative ways; our practice can lead, over time, to a heightened appreciation of the wondrous beauty of being. Yogic practice is, at bottom, a deeply creative approach that allows the ordinary mind to discover that significance fills every experience; every experience can become a work of art.

The arts play an important role in Western culture. In a world that seems to have been disenchanted by the rise of technical knowledge, art gives access to dimensions of feeling that cannot easily be expressed in rational language. Works of art encourage us to look deeply at the physical world, and see it as a manifestation of sacred energies. Without this precious embodiment, without manifestation, no work of art can exist. Art depends on the body, but at the same time it also reveals the body's hidden beauty.

The great siddhas were artists without a canvas; their way of being in the world was their masterpiece, and even their most ordinary gestures and expressions could conduct creativity. As we practice Kum Nye, we can do this in our own ways. Through these simple exercises, if we practice with sincerity, we can develop creativity as a way of being.

A dance of space

As we exercise, as we harmonize, we open up. Embodied knowledge engages at all levels, touching tissues, cells, perhaps even the finest subatomic particles, as awareness descends to the bottom of the senses. In the depths, we can discover that we are truly united. Here there is no distinction of self and other; no pointing "to," no love "of" that discriminates and separates into good and bad, desired and avoided. At this deep level, awareness expands into bliss.

Body and mind coordinating, senses in harmony, free to express a myriad of characters and potentials, we begin to experience our human embodiment as a kind of choreography, a dance of space.

We know that on an atomic level, we are all connected; but we are also connected with space. In the West, we tend to think of bodies in space, as if space were just an inert container for matter. But the heart of our being opens to space. Moving deeper and deeper within the body, we become united with the openness of space. We are not just dancing in space; perhaps we are the way space dances.

CHAPTER FOUR

JOY OF DANCING

*The Kum Nye dance expresses sacred knowledge in motion;
it hints at what it might mean to embody deep realization. This
dance, arising from the heart of space, is space's reply to the
unspoken question of our embodiment, the mystery of our being.
Here and now, space is dancing us.*

Body touching mind

Even when we are not actively practicing Kum Nye, we can work in a Kum Nye way with experience, becoming conscious of physical and emotional habits, and allowing our ordinary thoughts, feelings and movements to become our teachers.

Western thinking on the nature of human being has divided up body and mind into separate realms. Because of this legacy of thought, we might be inclined to view the work of yoga as a joining up of two discrete entities, "body" and "mind." Yet the subtle harnessing of yogic practice is a process by which intimate relations are revealed. The closer we look, the harder it is to find a firm separation of body and mind; at the finer perceptual levels, there may be only a conceptual discrimination that is held in place by long tradition and individual habit. Because of our limited concepts of body and mind, we might miss the energy at play within us; but this playful life energy does not keep within the strict lines delineated by our cultural and linguistic assumptions about the shape of the world.

The body's refreshment has great power to refresh the mind. Kum Nye may seem like exercises performed by and for the body, but each exercise, each movement, is reflected in the play of subtle energy; the release of tension frees up this energy and lets it move naturally. Body and mind together dance and play.

Associations and connections

Certain sounds are comforting; certain smells can evoke complex memories. Through sights, odors, flavors, we can experience other times, and revisit earlier periods of our lives. All of us have experienced a memory-association when we taste a certain food or hear a certain song. But the associations may be more interwoven and complex than we realize. Perhaps all sensations are dense with associations, some obvious, some more subtle.

We can start with a smell that has a strong association for us—the fragrant steam rising from a cup of jasmine tea; the smoky smell of new asphalt; the freshness of a wind blowing in from the ocean. We can see how these odors do not stand alone, but connect with other sense impressions: the ocean breeze is cool and crisp, and we can feel the moisture in it; the asphalt gives just a little under our feet; the tea feels silky on our tongue. The senses are working together to produce these experiences.

We can trace associations broadly in space and time; a smell does not just remind us of earlier smells, but can evoke an entire felt world of sense-experience. The smell of new paint has the power to conduct us back in time to a childhood home, or our first experiences living on our own as adults. Certain experiences show these connections and associations more clearly, but closer study of the texture of experience suggests that these connections inform all our sense impressions with subtle comparisons, connotations, and memories that flash through us almost too quickly to perceive.

Both in practice and in our daily lives, we can explore our experiences, sensing the way even a brief glance down at a shirt cuff or the sensation of the keyboard beneath our fingers is linked to a matrix of prior experience. How powerful this subliminal influence on our perceptions might be!

Sensitivity and appreciation

Sensitivity is often conceived as a reaction to something. Our skin prickles in response to a stimulus; our pupils dilate in response to light. Emotionally, we may feel as if every experience affects us strongly; a word spoken can alter our feelings for hours. Sensitivity understood in this way becomes a kind of vulnerability; being sensitive can seem like a burden. But perhaps this is too limited a definition; perhaps sensitivity is not what we think it is. Perhaps it is possible to have exquisite sensitivity without getting knocked off-balance. If we look closely at what we call our sensitivity, we can see that our loss of balance has something to do with our reactions. We reach for things we want; we draw back from things we do not want. This constant oscillation keeps us from ease. Yet when we begin to realize the extent to which our experience is colored by these movements, we get a fresh opportunity to explore other dimensions of feeling.

Moments of appreciation can help us practice sensitivity without grasping or avoiding experience. We can find this appreciation when we stop to consider even the simplest things. They can move us so deeply: the gleam of sunlight on green grass, the smell of food cooking—all these ordinary blessings can become sources of inspiration. Feeling a cool breeze on our face, we do not have to try to catch the wind; we can allow it to play out and follow its nature. We can appreciate the soft touch, and do not need to fear its gradual easing into stillness.

At first, we may feel that certain experiences can be appreciated and inhabited in this way, but others cannot. This kind of sensitivity sounds marvelous in theory, the rational mind argues, but in reality it is difficult to do anything but crave the things we feel we need, or seek to avoid the things that seem likely to bring trouble. Painful sensations still cause us to tense up; freezing cold or burning heat will cause us to flinch away. Persuaded by these reasonable arguments, we may consider our craving and aversion to be natural reactions, and we divide our experience up accordingly. Yet as we get more familiar with the internal qualities of our experience, our initial reactions begin to change. Eventually, even more challenging sensations can be encompassed by sensitive, open awareness. A toothache, for example, does not have to be an occasion for panic; the pain experience does not have to cause the mind to shut down.

As wise and sensitive practitioners, we do not want to let a situation harmful to the body keep on developing; we do our best to take care of ourselves. But we are not driven by our fearful associations with pain to take foolhardy actions— or to avoid necessary actions. In this way, true sensitivity is a key component of

∴

practical, working intelligence. Without fear, without craving, sensitivity grows finer; awareness expands. What is the thing being touched so sensitively? Could it be that craving and avoidance are reactions to a separation that does not really exist? Are we, finally, part of what we sense?

A hint of sweetness

Think of the way an intense flavor affects our bodies: it charges through us, stimulating our senses, dominating our attention. We have a similar reaction to strong bursts of emotion, not just anger or grief or fear but even seemingly positive emotions like excitement, or consuming passion. Like too much perfume in the air, the swooning intensity becomes all we are able to detect; when it passes, we may feel blank and numb. But working with subtler, milder sensations, we can awaken deeper awareness. It can start with just a hint of beauty, like a cool breeze passing through a hot room, like a ray of light emerging out of clouds. We experience a quiet, unobtrusive, dawning awareness of sweetness, of nourishment. We may have to become more observant to detect this hint of sweetness. But we are not leaning on awareness, pushing to see or taste. Ordinary concepts of effort may not serve us well in this case. It is as if we were trying to hold a dandelion puff in our hands: if we grasp it too firmly, it will quickly disperse its seed.

We can take an exploratory response instead, reserving judgment on what we are perceiving. A judgment, like "this is sweet," finishes off our engagement; we have determined what we are dealing with, and we then put it down to move on to the next thing that needs to be identified. We do not have to judge or even identify our experiences. We can dwell with the sky, receiving its many colors, as it gradually changes from light blue to gold and orange to dusky purple. There are colors within colors, colors that have never had names. If we are patient, we can sense these subtle colors, in the world, in ourselves.

Encouraging gentleness

Once we start to get a feeling for the quality of awareness that seems to give the best results, we can apply this calmer, more casual sensitivity, this subtler kind of observation, at finer and finer levels.

Breathing lightly, we make contact with the depths of the breath. With soft eyes, we touch the depths of seeing. We can make direct contact with light, something we don't always notice, because we are too busy seeing the things around us with the aid of light. Hearing and smelling, touching and tasting may be the same. It may take time and patience to excavate them, but we can develop more and more knowledge of our senses, our experience, through gentleness. And, gentleness can take us to depths of feeling that forcing cannot reach.

Developing flexibility

The gradual approach of Kum Nye works with real-world manifestations and expressions, softening and easing them toward smoothness. This step-by-step approach does not reject the world presented to us by our senses. Instead, Kum Nye massages these structures, slowly opening them up, expanding the range of motion available. Tensions and blockages may not vanish in a puff of smoke, but gradually they do change, like wax getting softer in the hand. With practice, qualities of experience that seem like hard realities become more malleable.

As we develop greater flexibility in our senses and responses, breathing can be our teacher. As we take in air, our lungs gently expand. The feeling of air going in, of the lungs opening, accommodating, is a direct, nourishing experience of our flexibility. The feeling of air freely going out as we exhale—that too is flexibility.

Experience shows us that the body can improve its flexibility with even a little practice; but we can contact this kind of flexibility directly within feeling. The flexibility of the body, flexibility of feeling, and flexibility of perception are all connected. Gradually, we begin to develop even deeper flexibility; the "I" itself begins to soften up. Even if the body seems, from our ordinary perspective, to have limits to its flexibility, the mind has no such constraints. Awareness is infinitely

∴

flexible; expanding and condensing, embracing and accommodating, it remains vibrant and joyful, full of life.

Softening intensity

The body is capable of a gamut of expressions. In a short span of time, we can experience joy, love, grief, and anger. Perplexity, frustration, and deep confusion are performances enacted by our bodies and senses. Even the disjointed feeling we experience when mind and body are disconnected is finally just another way of operating, another manifestation of energy.

Painful sensations; the numbness of blocking out the world; the heat of anger; the high drama of personal outrage; the pathos of loneliness: all these forms of emotional turmoil are active expressions of body energies. Some of them may seem harsh and strange, but ultimately they are part of us; they are ways, roles that our body and our sensations have learned to perform. With prolonged, direct experience of the unity that underlies these varied intensities, we can learn to soften them up. We can learn to massage tense situations internally, working directly with feeling and breath to tame and gentle the wary quality of our awareness.

Without controlling the breath, we can allow it to move through us, relaxing the belly, the heart, and the throat. We pay attention in a gentle way; there is no need to fight. Breath moves smoothly, filling and nourishing each cell as we inhale, tapering off almost imperceptibly as we exhale. Although they can seem sharp and stark, our sense-experiences, too, are moving, changing, filling us through and through, and gradually dispersing.

Breathing, we allow our awareness of the sensation to expand, noting how it ripples outward, shifting its tone over time. Fierce anger rises, peaks, and settles down; amusement may come up suddenly in its wake, leaving a trail of shining bubbles as it flows through us. It is all subject to change; it is all gradually changing. As we allow ourselves to feel the great breadth and depth of our sensations, they lose their discreteness, merging with one another at their outer edges. The stormy weather ebbs away, leaving us in a quiet sea.

.·:·.

Breathing alchemy

Breathing helps us recognize our intimate connection with the world around us, for the air we breathe is not just going in and out of our lungs, but unites with and revitalizes the body, working within our cells to help convert the food we eat into usable forms of energy. But breathing energy plays many subtle roles within the body, affecting our spirits and minds as well; it coordinates the relationships of our embodiment.

Breath manifests the state of mind and body; it can show us clearly how we are feeling. Ragged breathing, shallow breathing, harsh breathing—when the breath catches on something, we can feel it as a kind of obstruction in the throat, or in the chest.

When we are preoccupied, anxious, unable to let go of thoughts and feelings, it becomes hard to breathe, as if the space for breath is already full; tension can reduce our lung capacity and leave us breathing shallowly. This, in turn, increases our anxiety, and a feedback loop is created. But breathing practice can teach us how to use the breath to turn this situation around.

As breath moves through our bodies, it refines, extracts, purifies, and alchemizes. Breathing acts like a wire transmission, sending energy through the nadis, the subtle channels of the body. When we pay attention to our breath, we soften up, becoming more receptive to this gentle, penetrating, non-stop energy transmission. A constant cascade of fresh energy renews our tissues and sharpens our minds. Breath travels everywhere, visiting every point in the body; breathing practice can carry our awareness to subtle and secret parts of the body, inner tissues and chemical structures that would otherwise be inaccessible to us.

Breathing exercises activate the transmission powers of the breath, allowing it to be a means of communication; energy travels from node to node, chakra to chakra, lighting up every part of the body. As we learn to refine our own breathing, it regulates our energy flow, allowing our tensions to ease.

In the yogic tradition, breathing practices could lead to profound self-mastery, even altering the yogi's body down to the cellular level. Gradually, as breathing expands awareness, ordinary ways of inhabiting the body and experiencing the world begin to change. Through breathing, it may be possible to create a very different way of being embodied.

Releasing the pose

As we practice, we can take time to notice our own gestures, how we hold ourselves, catching a glimpse of the image we produce for others, the image we produce for ourselves. As we work more closely with the positions and gestures of Kum Nye, we may find that we are holding a pose even when we think we are being natural. Posing can have many purposes. We pose for a picture or a photograph, presenting a certain appearance to be looked at. But posing can also mean dissembling; we might pose as more knowledgeable than we actually are. This aspect of posing goes back to posing as performance, a form of acting. But just as the actor is different from his role, we, too, can begin to loosen up our identification with our habitual postures, our posing as ourselves.

We can pay attention casually, throughout the day. Whether we are driving, sitting at a desk, preparing food, or working physically, we can begin to notice the poses and postures we take in our daily lives. What attitudes are we presenting when we clench our hands, hunch our shoulders, or tighten our jaws? As we explore and begin to let go of our poses, we may discover that we are assuming not just physical but emotional and mental postures, frozen attitudes that manifest as rigidity of feeling, or a certain numbness. Just as we can relax our hands on the steering wheel, perhaps we can relax some of our ideas and beliefs, and some of our habitual emotional states. What if all these emotions that grip us so strongly are just poses, like the frozen postures of Kabuki actors? Releasing the tension that holds these poses in place also releases feeling. It allows blocked emotions a chance to melt.

When we begin to penetrate the posing, posing itself is liberated: it can become a medium of expression. Many poses are possible; we need not be confined only to certain modes of being. We get a chance to recognize that our experiences, which seem so solid and distinct, are expressions of a deeper unity; their characters become translucent. We begin to sense that this is just one way for the world to manifest. Finally, gradually waking up, shaking off our numbness, we may begin to tap our beaks against the eggshell of our most fundamental posing—our "being."

Characters and performances

The softness and warmth of the wool blanket we tuck around us when we get cold; the three sweet, descending notes of a blackbird's song; the rich amber color of the tea we pour; the clarifying smell of eucalyptus; all of these experiences have unique and distinct characters. Yet their distinctiveness, their appearance to us as real phenomena, is due to their being part of a complex regime of perception and meaning, a shifting lattice of differences and distinctions. Just as words receive their meanings through a process of comparison and contrast with other words, other meanings, the characters of experience emerge from a similar network of relationships.

The word "character" also refers to a figure in a story or play. Our sensory impressions, our perceptions, our feelings, our thoughts, our fantasies and plans—even our concepts—perhaps they are characters. When we consider our experiences as expressive characters, it changes the impact of what we experience. Characters communicate, express, and perform: we call this the nature of experience. Characters have distinctive shapes and forms. Yet they have no substance; for substance itself is a character, a manifestation of a fundamentally open being.

The characters of our experience can remind us that there is something playful about our embodiment, our manifestation of sacred energy. Rough and tough, or soft and gentle; perhaps we are capable of playing many roles, expressing many characters. Seen in this light, experience can become play, a pure and pliable medium of creative expression. As we practice Kum Nye, we get a glimpse behind the scenes; the performer is playing itself. It peeks out from behind the mask and whispers, "Hey, this is an act."

Ripples in time

Intellectually, we can appreciate that the drama of our emotions might be a kind of illusion, a passing state, just as we know that ice or hail are manifestations of H_2O. We can perceive a similarity between the planet's weather systems, and the weather of the heart. But we tend to experience our emotions as things that happen to us—storms that come upon us suddenly, and must simply be endured.

.:.

We attribute the same unquestioned reality to our sensations and feelings. Our senses, such as our eyes and ears act as gatekeepers, noticing ripples in feeling and identifying each one as a distinct state. Our senses provide the feedbacks to the mind that produce the unified fabric of experience. It all seems perfectly consistent and solid; it is a very convincing story. Everything we perceive, both inside and outside ourselves, seems to have a distinct identity. Yet those different characters are a function of a ceaseless processing and comparing of flows of sensation whose true nature may be hard to define.

We can see an analogous situation in the world of matter and energy in which we exist. The objects of our experience play certain fixed roles in the world of our understanding, but we have learned that these physical manifestations are temporary expressions of energy. Like matter itself, sensations seem to have distinct identities. Hard is not soft; hot is not cold. Yet sensations are constantly shifting, changing over time. Noticing the way our fingertips rest lightly on a surface, we find that contact is constantly changing.

We can get in close touch with the rippling of our oceanic experience by heightening our awareness of time. Patiently, sensitively noticing these changes as they occur, we can begin to perceive our sensations, our feelings, even our thoughts, as movements, ripples in a soft and subtle medium; they no longer seem quite like static states. As we look more closely, we may notice ripples emerging from ripples— filling the apparently blank spaces and times when we supposedly have nothing going on. How far in space, in time, might these ripples extend?

Waves of expression

There is a majestic quality to the ocean waves; in their heights and depths, they manifest grandeur, drama, but also a kind of purity. Water rises and falls; energy travels in waves. The many characters of our thoughts, our feelings, the innumerable shadings of our physical experience, are, in their own fashion, waves. When we truly begin to understand this, we need not fear their power.

We say that high tide is different than low tide, but this difference may only be a matter of comparisons. In a way, each of these characters is a ratio: it is an

.:.

amalgam of sensations, of paired opposites juxtaposed within us at a level just below conscious awareness.

What happens if we treat our experiences as expressions of energy? We begin to experience our movements and gestures as waves, ripples. But perhaps our thoughts, too, are waves; and perhaps even our most rigid responses, habits, and beliefs are actually in subtle motion.

Emotional states manifest as tension that inhibits the breath. But breath itself manifests the waving, the rippling of nature. As breath rises and falls, we can fearlessly experience its many expressions, recognizing for ourselves that these seeming obstacles are just waves—fundamental openness appearing for a brief moment in a certain shape and form.

Supported by water

The education we receive, the compulsion to obey the rules of society, the definitions and distinctions of language, and the pros and cons that set up our conceptual thinking all serve to create tension that can affect the clarity of our thoughts, dull the vividness of our senses and feelings, and bind our bodies into frozen, uncomfortable postures. Like a persistent, low-grade virus, tension is ever-present within and around us.

We may be so accustomed to living in this state that we have stopped noticing the extent to which we are hampered; we no longer realize that gradually, almost imperceptibly, we may have lost our ability to embody joy.

Kum Nye's gentle attention to the intimate details of our experience can unlock these frozen states. Concentrating lightly, we exhale, allowing each movement of our bodies to encourage and extend the flow of the breath. Each shift of position can release tension, melting the blockages we have been keeping in our feet, our joints, our backs, our bellies, necks and shoulders. Moving freely, we can untangle the knots in the stomach, soften the obstruction in the throat, and uncover the tension hidden in our faces and behind our eyes. In time, these movements can release not only physical tension, but the subtler tension of sensing, thinking, and feeling. We let go, exhale, rejoice, release. Releasing becomes ease.

As we continue, eventually we can treat all of yogic practice as a continuous release of tension, conducting us to greater and greater ease. Ultimately, we are not just practicing one exercise, one pose at a time. Swimming has individual strokes, distinctive motions—but swimming itself is a smooth, continuous movement through the water. Our gestures gradually acquire this connected quality as we practice: body movements become a kind of floating in ease.

When we go swimming, water is our partner—if we rely on its support, our movements become completely relaxed. When we practice Kum Nye, feeling supports us like water. Our movements ease up tensions, as pain, fear, and resistance, even identity, are released. Ease expands, extends; as we float in feeling, thoughts, senses and movements become calm. Movement itself becomes floating relaxation, a natural expression of energy.

As we practice the movements and gestures of Kum Nye, and as we move through our daily lives, breathing can help us to develop this free-floating quality. If we are subtly holding resistance or tension, if we are experiencing pain, we can use this technique. Each time a movement changes, we can exhale, releasing tension. As tensions are released, we realize that what seemed like obstacles can become our friends. Our bodily experience, our sensations, thoughts and feelings, cradle us as water cradles the swimmer.

Un-fixing ourselves

We may be unwitting contributors to our tension. Our movements, our attitudes— our very attempts to relax—can tighten up our bodies. As soon as this tension is created, we lose access to the healing qualities of breath energy; this energy begins to stick here and there, locking up in tight corners inside us. We focus on the tension, and it intensifies; fixing our gaze on our problems, we find them getting worse. This intense gaze is what is often called awareness in the West; it may appear objective, but it has the side-effect of crystallizing what we look at, locking it into position. This is not the same kind of calm and curious attention we pay when we are sitting back, watching. We are right up in front, the active agent, the one who seeks to do the fixing.

The innocent student says, "I tried to relax, but I couldn't manage it, sorry—I got panicky. I'm not focusing hard enough on improvement, I forgot—I'm still intense—I'm still tight—I don't know how to change." Identifying faults, owning mistakes: we are told this is the right thing to do, but by doing so, we can strengthen their hold over us and reinforce their power. The "I" is fixed, stuck in place with the flaws it has pointed out.

Once we are stuck with our mistakes, we may rebel against our own instruction, talk back to ourselves: "I don't feel like doing this! I've had enough!" The dialogue goes back and forth; but there is no opportunity for a new conversation, no soothing quality to the interaction. This does not fix the problem. This fixing fixes us in place, causing tension to build. Even our problems are fixed into position. But this is not surprising. How, under such circumstances, could they possibly be released?

When we loosen up, let go of our instructions, and spontaneously embrace our experience, gradually our self-confidence grows. We may not need to fix ourselves after all; perhaps what we really need is to un-fix ourselves. We learned how to be worried, how to be upset; now it is time to un-learn, to wipe the slate clean.

Correction and change

Often, we correct ourselves, and call that practice, or refining the self. In order to learn a skill, critique and correction are important; but there is a difference between making a correction and performing in the present moment. The act of correction depends on memory, judgment, and projection; we look at our activity as it compares to a certain baseline. To the extent that our activity matches the pattern, we call that action correct. But correction in the ordinary sense presupposes separation. The corrector is separate from the correct-ee; and both are separate from the ideal, the template used by the corrector-self.

In the act, as it is really taking place, there is only doing; in that moment of pure activity, there is no room for correction. When we make changes from a desire to improve, we can remember that the moment of action is innocent of all judgment, all comparison, and all correction.

We are one with our bodies; this understanding is essential to unlocking the transformative potential of Kum Nye. It is important to treat our bodies with kindness, for they are not objects we possess, but intimately ourselves.

Befriending all experience

In our zeal to improve, we may treat our habits, our negativities, our weaknesses as the enemy; but when we take such an attitude, we end up fighting ourselves. As we study our experience through Kum Nye, we discover that we need not make enemies of any part of our experience. The qualities of our experience are all emerging from constant relation and interaction with one another and with space; an intricate dance is taking place within us, an animated conversation with many participants is being held. These ever-changing combinations give rise to sensations, feelings, habits, and concepts—including the concept of "self." Awareness itself is not separate from these interactions, but part of the conversation, emerging from and contributing to its endless unfolding. Consciousness trained by Kum Nye practice can engage directly with regimes of thoughts, senses, and emotions, fostering positive interactions.

As we practice, we are not monitoring, dictating, or deal-making, but gently befriending. Like a gifted host or hostess who makes every guest feels at home, we can subtly, almost casually, integrate and harmonize all aspects of our experience. Gradually, what we once perceived as a distraction becomes part of our practice. The noise of passing cars or construction outside—even the voices of people around us—these things are included, welcomed into our experience. When they are greeted kindly, and accepted as part of what is taking place, they lose their sharp, harsh edges, and show us other sides. The hum of machinery can take us deeper into calmness; the voices of our fellow human beings can wake us up.

Experiencing this deep camaraderie with ourselves and our environment, we may discover we are more connected physically, better grounded emotionally, and more aware of how we relate. It is as if we are learning how to shake hands warmly and confidently with everything we experience: when we keep this friendly spirit, we find ourselves less likely to collide with the world around us. We can hold physical objects with the right amount of firmness, and provide soothing contact to our fellow living creatures.

This is Kum Nye as friendship: Kum (sKu) means body or substance, and Nye (mNye) means a process that encourages a friendly co-existence. Yogic practice helps us to join the ongoing conversation in a new way; we can see it as the art of making friends with all experience.

The present moment

We are beings with bodies; our lives unfold in time, and we inhabit each moment. Supposedly, we live in the present—yet so many of us feel as if we are missing out on the present moment, as if we are missing in some crucial way from our own lives. Perhaps what is missing is awareness; awareness is not in touch, so we cannot fully embody the sacred energy of the present moment. When our awareness is tangled up in memories, fantasies and projections, we can end up locked out of our own lives, in a perpetual state of longing for something real. How, then, can we cultivate being-present? How do we accomplish this—what do we need to do? Perhaps we do not need to do anything at all.

Certain yogic traditions use awareness of breathing as a tool for remaining in the present moment, but this method presents certain challenges to our goal-oriented perspective. If we put too much effort into breathing, it is difficult to relax the breath, and difficult to open up to our own being-present. Striving for a goal or ideal of embodied presence paradoxically makes it harder for awareness to open up to the present moment; it is preoccupied with striving, too busy chasing a state that has been pre-defined as "not happening yet," or "not achieved yet."

We do not need to make the present moment the goal of our practice. If we can let presence be, relaxation comes naturally, and we pass effortlessly through the obstructions created by our conceptual thinking. The present moment opens, ocean-wide.

Penetrating experience

The texture of ordinary life can be hard to discern. We seem to move quickly from event to event, from sensation to sensation, and it can be difficult to recall how we got from one to another. In the midst of our day, we can suddenly find ourselves angry, or dreamy, or deeply worried, or blank and confused. We experience these states vividly, yet somehow we are too busy, too pressed for time, to perceive how they occurred. Often, they appear to us as faits accomplis, finished products that do not seem to have any history at all. Kum Nye helps us learn how to penetrate our experience; as we practice, we can see more clearly how our sensations, our feelings, and our thoughts arise.

The productions of our experience offer us an ever-renewed opportunity to develop this awareness, for each seemingly finished product—each sensation, each thought, each feeling—is an ongoing show being hosted by our embodiment, a marvelous piece of theater unfolding in space and time. We can cultivate greater sensitivity to the regimes that govern our experience—the production company that underwrites the ongoing show we call being ourselves.

We can begin to explore the depths of our sensations by concentrating on simple activities like washing dishes, drinking tea, or eating a snack. Who knew that eating an apple could have such reverberations through our experience? The mingling of taste and smell; the evocative shape, the skin's smooth surface; the thoughts and comparisons, tiny flashes of anxiety, the memories of other moments, other apples combine and ramify. A single taste of sweetness seems to open up wider and wider dimensions as our awareness becomes more refined.

As we learn more and more about the way our experience is produced, experience gains in richness. Pleasure lasts longer; even uncomfortable sensations begin to yield surprisingly supportive qualities, as we identify and release our own resistance to feeling.

When we practice Kum Nye in this way, it becomes more than a set of exercises or ideas. It becomes a mode of inquiry, a space in which we are free to notice the mounting of the production, discovering the subtle operations of our senses, and the profound effects of language and culture upon the ways of being we normally take for granted.

The operations of our sense faculties affect everything about human life; like gateway guardians, they are the parts of us that negotiate with the outside world. Kum Nye helps us get to know the textures of sense-experience, and to discover what creates these textures—what circumstances and forces help to produce their distinctive qualities. We can imagine the five sense faculties as ushers: they conduct us to our seats, positioning human being within a lattice composed of physical conditions, cultural restraints, and personal history. How do these ushers do their work? Can we see just where we are being seated in the theater of space?

Opening feeling

We may understand intellectually that existence is fully open, merged with space, but our experience seems to be full of real objects, real circumstances, and real situations challenges.

Kum Nye is a gradual approach that works with the grain of experience, using our human condition, with its linear time, physical objects, and relationships and connections, as a sacred vehicle of transformation. Kum Nye begins with our ordinary expectations—that time flows forward, that bodies are solid, that cause and effect exist—and gently opens our minds to new experiences.

The methods of Kum Nye allow us to move at a pace that is more comfortable for the ordinary mind, introducing us bit by bit to this openness. Layer by layer, little by little, our sense perceptions, thoughts and feelings can be transformed. Like a lotus with hundreds of petals, each sensation has subtle gradations and shifts within it. Yet the deeper we go, the more we relax into the sensation, the more open and spacious the sensation itself becomes. Sensation may be like an onion with many layers—but this onion gets larger as each layer is removed. We can explore these layers by working with a single exercise over time. Over the course of a few weeks or months, we may see different responses to the same exercise.

We can take the same approach to open up the depth and complexity of a single moment of feeling, gently penetrating the layers of a single sensation. When we massage the body's tissues, we can feel how our response to the touch of our hand gradually opens up: the feeling changes as tension is released. In the same way, we can massage our perceptions, our feelings, memories, and thoughts. We can explore the subtle layers of our response to a single color, how that color is woven into the fabric of our sense of self.

Concepts of sensation

In the West, concept and sensation are often treated as opposites. This is a mark of a deep-seated division between mind and body that organizes, in profound ways, how we relate to experience. According to our habitual categories, sensation belongs to the body; concepts belong to the mind. Yet when we look closely, we can see that the things we call sensations are themselves conceptual entities. When sensations are placed in cognitive boxes, they become states. States are knowable objects, firmly mapped territories in our inner geography. We navigate by our states; our belief in them helps them to keep their positions, upholding the regular operations of ordinary experience. In this way, a state can actually be anchored in place by language—and can become an anchor for feeling, weighing us down.

Pain is an illuminating example. Once it has been identified as "pain," subject to comparisons with "pleasure," firmly in its conceptual box, pain is a no-change agent, driving us along in a continuation of the sense regime. In the grip of our definitions of pain, we are helpless to act creatively. We all know what pain is, yet as it is being felt, at certain moments pain can open up into sensations that are harder to classify. When we gently penetrate feeling, opening up layer by layer, even pain may begin to change. As we explore our experience, allowing sensations to develop and flow more freely, we can begin to loosen up our sensation-concepts.

Stretching, if we are unused to it, can be at first a little painful. But if we stretch very kindly and gradually, without forcing anything, we can actually feel that pain change its tone, become something other than pain. We can become sensitive to the moment when our sensations begin to shade away from known states, and become unknown territory. Increasing flexibility of body, of sensation and of thought emerges as the known feeling states, the sensations we identify, lose their rigid identifications. As we open to the full dimensionality of our sensations, we unlock the cognitive boxes that give sensations their ordinary, habitual shape.

At a deeper level, the fundamental idea that sensations are things experienced by selves—this concept of sensation-hood that underpins the wild variety of our experiences—begins to soften up. Slowly, we start to shed layers of separateness from our experience.

Is it possible that all sensations communicate at bottom? Perhaps all of them, without exception, have the power to conduct us beyond ourselves to the same place-less place—the open field.

Exploring tension

We are accustomed to perceiving tension as an ill, something to be avoided; but we may not have taken a close look at what our tension is, what its ingredients are, and how it came to exist. Tension is often defined as a physical state of constriction or restriction; it hardens muscle tissues and rigidifies joints. In the ordinary way, we characterize tension as a reaction to something; it has a cause. Something bad happens, and we tense up. Or we think something bad is going to happen, and we tense up in anticipation. Tension hardens the barrier: Keep out! But tension cannot protect us from harm. Tension itself is harmful. It hurts to feel, and it hurts to maintain. But this may only be the final stage of tension's expression; if we look more closely, we might discover that this quality of bracing against experience arose in the mind before we tightened up our muscles.

As we explore our sense-experience, we may begin to detect subtler forms of tension. There is the tension of being aware of something: grasping and aversion are both tension states. We can trace tension in our fixed patterns, habits, and operations. Finally, and most subtle of all, is the tension involved in holding together subjective identity.

We begin to see the tension involved in holding on, bracing against, obeying, and disobeying: being ourselves—being selves, with all the obligations self-hood entails. We tense up to protect ourselves; but this separate self is itself an expression of tension. In the end, tension may be a manifestation of separation; for when we relax our insistent separateness, our tensions begin to release.

Resting on the balance point

At the surface level of experience, we seem to find much activity. But just as ripples disturb only the surface of the ocean, the deeper we move into feeling, the quieter it becomes.

As we learn to deepen relaxation, the body gets more juice; it is nourished by joy, and set free from distraction. This joy rises up freely within our field of being; it requires nothing apart from us in order to flourish. Tensions melt away; we settle into calmness, not separate and alone, but part of a whole, at one with our environment. Releasing tension, we reach a moment of exquisite balance, a resting point of ease.

Inner garden of experience

A garden that is thriving offers us beauty all year round. It shows us riches of color, scent and texture: the glitter of droplets in summer as birds play in the sprinklers, red leaves on green grass in the autumn, cool grays and greens in winter, a rain of flower petals on the spring breeze. Our ordinary understanding is that we must look at the garden to experience this kind of beauty. But the garden lives inside of us. The beauty we perceive is part of us.

We may have noticed that when we experience fulfillment and pleasure, we have a completely different kind of mind than we do under circumstances of suffering. When we feel calm and secure, thoughts do not torment us; even challenging situations seem less daunting, and our comfort zone expands. We feel a greater tolerance for the people and things around us. Food tastes better, and we seem to get more rest when we sleep.

Relatively few of us realize that this joyful mind, open and curious, peaceful and accommodating, can appear within us at any time. Until we understand that our experience is a garden we can cultivate, we are stuck with whatever circumstance has sown within us. The desolation we sometimes feel lays waste to our interior spaces. Worry grows like a strangling weed, choking off all our other feelings and sensations. Our preoccupations grow to monstrous heights, while our more fragile and subtle sense-experiences wither from lack of attention.

The soil of the mind is extraordinarily fertile. It will accept and foster a startling range of experiences, joyful and terrible. But once we have really penetrated the structure of our sense-experience, really seen our own regimented thinking at work, really experienced our feelings as ripples expanding in openness, the chain that binds our inward responses to our outward circumstances is broken. Nothing obligates us to suffer. There is no need to follow the prescriptions of our regimes.

When we truly recognize that our experience is fundamentally open and flexible, we are free to respond creatively. As we become masters of our own experience, we can re-plant the gardens of our minds. We can rekindle the joy of a past experience, allowing its energy to mingle with and transform the quality of the present moment.

All the joy, all the wonder we have ever known is still available to us; it is part of us, part of our cells. These experiences are not just faded memories, pressed flowers whose ghostly shapes we keep in our conscious minds—they are seeds. Sown within the present moment, they can flower again and again.

Gestures

At times, we may associate movement and change with sloppiness and incorrectness. If it's changing, it can't be pinned down; how can it be properly categorized and defined? We may have inherited this attitude from the operations of language, which cannot function without clear delineations between words. The world, seen through the lens of meaning, boils down to categories: "Yes, it is" or "no, it isn't." Softening our categories, opening our judgments, we begin to experience motion as free expression.

While there is a strong spirit of empirical observation and experimentation in Kum Nye, there is no need to translate that into a rigid or nit-picking approach that insists on perfection in the details. In fact, true precision—of a pitcher throwing a ball, of a dancer leaping and landing, of an archer releasing an arrow—is an expression of complete relaxation.

∵

As we practice, it is helpful to cultivate a curious, adventurous spirit. The exercises we use are tools for exploration, and the territory is truly new to us. We do not need to produce static, picture-perfect copies of positions, or rote-accurate movements. Indeed, we can think of these exercises as gestures.

Gestures are natural and spontaneous expressions of feeling. In animated conversation, we talk with our hands; in moments of deep affection, we embrace our loved ones; in unscripted happiness, we dance. We can see this relaxed beauty everywhere in the natural world, in the way a bird launches itself into the sky, the way a flower opens. Organic and inevitable, each gesture takes place in its own time, its own way. These gestures are unique. They cannot be repeated, for their beauty and appropriateness are in tune with this precise moment, this precise place in space.

Body of knowledge

Kum Nye gives us a new way to understand what it means to be familiar with, or aware of, one's body. Practice begins to give rise to a very different picture: we begin to see that awareness is not necessarily awareness of something. Instead, we find that awareness is intimacy: we discover that we are intimately sensing flows, fields, relations. The sensing perceiver, too, may not occupy a hard and fast position; when we make contact, we connect, and that flowing, floating quality of our experience becomes part of our sense of self. We begin to sense that energy is making contact with energy.

As energy unites with energy, another kind of consciousness can develop; a new awareness is free to emerge. Ordinary conceptual understanding is profoundly changed, for the basic context—the idea that the world is an object "out there" that can be known by a perceiver "in here"—has been transformed by direct experience.

The body's movements are manifestations of awareness; the body bodies forth knowledge beyond any concepts. The gestures of a realized yogi are not expressions of understanding; the expression is the understanding. There is no about-ness to this embodied knowledge; it is not a collection of information about anything.

We understand this kind of knowledge well in practical terms, for it is connected to walking the talk, embodying insight. On a deeper level, knowledge itself is transformed. We find that knowledge is not a picture or an idea we keep in our heads—not an overview taken by the mind of the body. The body itself is aware, expressing knowledge. Energy touching energy: perhaps this is the substance of the body's expression, the medium of knowledge's manifestation.

Depth of purpose

The purpose of our life activity is important. In Kum Nye, the purpose that informs our practice affects what we take away from that practice. If our purpose is small or self-oriented, the knowledge we get from our experience will be small and self-oriented in turn. If our purpose is larger, deeper, it lifts the restrictions on what we are able to gain from our practice, and from our lives. The definition of Kum Nye as "body massage" suggests that its purpose is to transform the body, or to alter sensory experience. But as we explore these practices, we may begin to sense a greater potential.

In Tibet, yogic training was not undertaken lightly. Its purpose was to break open the sense regimes, the complex, tightly-bound networks of associations and repetitions that structure our experience, even at the level of perception. When the sense regimes are penetrated, it becomes possible to release the energy that powers insight and, ultimately, transformation. For insofar as we believe the stories of our regimes, insofar as we think that we are slaves, we are stuck in a trap of our own making. The yogic practitioners set out to open the trap. They sought to change the structure of the self, to crack the hard shell of experience, and get the nutritious kernel that is inside.

Yogic training can bring to light the importance of our expression of energy, our specific embodiment, our moment in time, giving us the knowledge that ultimately there may be a reason for our being here, for our undertaking this journey. When we take our lives seriously, when we consider the possibility that we have work to do on this planet, it changes the way we practice. Starting from the present moment, the sacred zero-point of our embodiment here and now, we can develop our own sense of purpose.

This purpose is as unique and individual as a fingerprint; like the depth of bodily knowledge, it cannot easily be codified, but it can be freely expressed, in movement and stillness, in gesture and act. What is Kum Nye's ultimate purpose? It might be to help us make direct contact with our own purpose, our part in the field of being.

The yogic path

Nowadays, it is hard to take the yogi road; while yoga forms abound in the West, real masters, real texts, real models, and real precedents are few. To follow the path requires discipline and patience. Living in the modern world, we have been conditioned to expect quick results, and may not know how to do the hard work the great yogic practitioners of the past undertook to unlock their inner potential.

The exercises of Kum Nye set clear goals, lay out methods to follow, and offer gentle, harmless ways to focus energy and attention. Although they may seem preliminary, if they are practiced with care, they can at the very least improve our well-being, enriching the soil of our experiences, strengthening our trust in our senses, and allowing us to access a deeper sense of our own aliveness.

Learning how to live within the deeper currents of feeling, we can sense the fundamental unity that gives rise to our individual experiences. Studying with the adventurous spirit of the yogis of old, we can learn for ourselves how to contact and rely upon this inner clarity.

The yogic path follows no formula. It cannot be replicated or duplicated—but it can be created anew by each practitioner in turn. As we continue to practice, we begin to cherish all of our experiences, and respect them as our teachers. We can see that the road stretches out in front of us; the path can take us to lands no one has explored yet, for each body, each experience is its own undiscovered country.

Sharing wholeness

The essence of Kum Nye is bliss. One of the dangers of the path is the possibility of becoming addicted to bliss. In India, bliss was considered the domain of the gods; Westerners, on the other hand, might recognize the quest for this state as "the pursuit of happiness." Life becomes a constant search for enjoyment, leisure and amusement; in the course of the hunt we may pursue the powerful bursts of pleasure afforded by certain foods and drugs or by sexual activity. Alternatively, we may retire into our fantasies, seeking refuge in the marvelous and seemingly imperishable creations of our minds.

These forms of stimulation do not last long, and in the end they are not very effective. They have the negative consequence of forcing us to chase continually in the highways and byways of our ordinary, conditioned sense-experiences for increasingly fugitive sensations of well-being; in the end, we come up empty.

Yogic practice appears to be precisely the opposite of this mad pursuit of pleasure. Yet even though we may be very sincere practitioners, if we become attached to the positive feelings our practice brings us, we are in danger of falling into this pursuit of happiness, which ultimately leads us back to the comparisons and judgments, the pros and cons, and the self-orientation that trap us in the sensation regimes.

Our search must take us further, beyond ordinary well-being, to the very bottom of sense-experience. Here, even our own pleasure reveals itself as part of something larger; our hearts open as we perceive our intimate connection to our surroundings. We begin to realize that compassion for others cannot be separated from this deep and growing awareness. The heart liberates us from addiction to the pleasure of our personal well-being, putting us in contact with a larger welfare, a larger joy. Health, ultimately, is wholeness; this wholeness encompasses all experience, without discrimination.

As we continue to make contact with this shared wholeness, the residual anxiety, the lingering fear of loss that drives us to take refuge in pleasurable experiences at last begins to dissolve. Then we are ready. We have tasted the real fruits of Kum Nye. Once we have touched the depths of sense-experience, tasted that unchangeable essence, and fully realized our basic openness, formal practice is not necessary. The beauty of being pours in on all sides; there is no need to go searching for it, to hoard the experience or fear its disappearance. This feeling takes over and gradually transforms the mind.

Our becoming whole is what frees us to become teachers and helpers, for sharing is built into our understanding; compassion and awareness are partners.

∴

Knowledge of yogic technique, or even knowledge of its higher purposes, is not enough; with this conceptual kind of knowledge, we can make some progress, but inwardly we are still bluffing, still not quite sure. When we have gained unshakeable confidence in wholeness, we cannot help but share our experience with others, for it shines in us, in our bodies, our minds, and our actions.

Dancing a mystery

Relaxation, release, opens our range of motion. It becomes possible to dance. Dancing is an expression of the body's joy, a gesture that transforms ordinary movement into art. Dance salvages our suffering, re-presents the characters of human experience, revealing it all as beautiful and meaningful.

In dance, the regimes of sense become artistic resources; the structures they have prescribed are no longer constricting. They are vibrating with life, fluid and ever-changing, rich with potential shape and form.

The yogi's dance expresses sacred knowledge in motion; it hints at what it might mean to embody deep realization. This dance, arising from the heart of space, is space's reply to the unspoken question of our embodiment, the mystery of our being. Here and now, space is dancing us.

THE GESTURES

The exercises presented in this volume belong to an esoteric tradition where instructions are transmitted orally in order to guarantee direct experience of the teaching and to protect its power and purity. The external forms of the postures can be described in writing and demonstrated through photographs for the interested reader, but to become a practitioner requires training with an authorized teacher, such as Arnaud Maitland.

TARTHANG TULKU

Approaching Kum Nye

Based on Tarthang Tulku's oral teachings to Western students at the Nyingma Institute in Berkeley, California in the early 1970s, the first book on Kum Nye in the West appeared in 1978 in two volumes entitled *Kum Nye Relaxation* Parts I and II. Thirty years later, in 2008, both volumes were integrated under the title *Kum Nye – a Tibetan Yoga. Kum Nye Relaxation* focused on loosening up the body and the embodiment by stimulating the flow of feeling through body, senses, and mind. Sitting, breathing, self-massage, postures, and movement exercises balance and integrate body and mind. An abundant vitality quickens in the body. Along the way, tension is released and the energies and intelligence of body and mind are integrated into a deep abiding calmness, like a quality of floating in space. As relaxation deepens, a subtle level of feeling opens like a lens, letting in more light and more comprehensive pictures of reality.

Tarthang Tulku Rinpoche's second Kum Nye book, *The Joy of Being*, published in 2006, introduced a new approach that aims to rebuild the inner architecture of the subtle body energy system while specifically focusing on opening the senses and relaxing the mind. This 'Kum Nye for the Mind' begins with refreshing the senses so that they can function as two-way channels and open into non-dual seeing, hearing, feeling, and thinking. Relaxing the labeling of experience in what is revealed as 'Speech Kum Nye' is pivotal in this approach. Through giving mind the space to be, new capabilities and qualities become accessible to us. We experience new sights, sounds, smells, tastes, and feelings. We gain access to a knowing that is truly ours.

Kum Nye Dancing

As Rinpoche writes in the introduction to this book, his third publication on Kum Nye, the movements and postures included here were introduced to community workers at an Odiyan temple plaza in 2008. Under the red skies of the sun setting over the Pacific Ocean, amid blazing winds, Rinpoche led his students deeper and deeper into the world of lama dancing. The postures and movements demanded expressive bodily gestures, dynamic and dramatic yet at the same time displaying a profound inner silence and quietude, and the conviction of being present in the present.

In *Kum Nye Dancing* you find no suggestions to develop relaxation, create balance, or promote integration. This book assumes that Nye (mNye) is already optimal and self-sustaining within you, and that Kum (sKu) is expansive and stable. The practitioner expresses unity of body and mind and begins to dance in space. Thus the seventy-six gestures in this book are presented in unvarnished terms that simply describe the gestures without engaging in details of how to direct energy, where to place emphasis, or what a particular gesture or sequence of gestures might mean. The left-hand pages offer descriptions of the gestures displayed in the photographs on the right-hand pages. Each description begins with a quote from the main text by Rinpoche. Many quotes might have referred to any of the other gestures; they are universal. May their timeless truth inspire you during your practice!

What you are invited to generate in yourself is the flexibility and openness to befriend all of your experience and express the openness of being. The postures and movements in themselves overcome all manner of hesitation, holding back, and resistance, making you ready to dance at all times.

It is recommended that you study and practice the first two Kum Nye books in depth, fully activating the Nye, before focusing on the gestures in Kum Nye Dancing. In this way you have the best chance of developing a deep knowledge of your individual embodiment, the specific expression of sacred energy called 'myself.'

Eight series

The gestures in Kum Nye Dancing are arranged in eight series, and it is recommended to begin with Series 1 and gradually build up to Series 7 before exploring the final series, examples of long dances. However, you may also choose a gesture from each series in order to build your own sequence for a long dance.

SERIES 1 - Seated gestures for being in the body and being present in space.

SERIES 2 - Gestures that stir and call forth the energies of the lower body energy centers, the power base, without which nothing can be established or sustained.

SERIES 3 - Gestures that bring you back to the ground, expressing the integration of grounding with lower body energies.

SERIES 4 - Gestures for the throat and upper body as managers of all internal and external communication.

SERIES 5 - Gestures that invoke new dimensions in space, displaying your growing level of participation and engagement in the union of left and right, up and down, and inner and outer.

SERIES 6 - Gestures that challenge you to utilize all inner and outer resources of energy and insight in fully engaging in the present.

SERIES 7 - Gestures showing creativity as a way of being.

SERIES 8 - A pictorial display of sample sets of dance postures and movements.

Bringing in rhythm

In Kum Nye dancing it is important to first become familiar with the gestures in their details. Once you feel at ease with the postures and movements, then it is time to bring in the rhythmic pulse that awakens the element of timing in you. You can begin to add rhythm by counting 1–2–3–4 either out loud or silently. Moving into the posture, performing each part of the movement, and releasing the posture all occur to the rhythm of four beats. For example, the arms move up to shoulder height to a count of four beats. The arms remain in the position for four beats, then move to the left to a count of four beats, remain there for four beats, and so on.

Sometimes it may feel appropriate to experiment with speeding up the rhythm, as in counting 1–2 to move into the gesture, or even just 1, and then holding the gesture for the same amount of time, so that the rhythm is distributed equally throughout the gesture.

Finally, as you develop the rhythmic movements in a particular sequence, you are ready to combine the gestures of your choice into a complete dance.

Sitting posture

The recommended sitting posture in Kum Nye is called The Seven Gestures. If you are physically unable to sit in the seven gestures, instead sit with the spine straight, breathing through nose and mouth with the tip of the tongue touching the upper palate.

The seven gestures are: (1) crossed legs, (2) the palms of the hands resting on the knees, (3) the back straight, (4) the chin slightly tucked in, (5) the mouth slightly open, (6) the tip of the tongue lightly touching the upper palate, (7) the eyes soft and open. In Kum Nye dancing, the eyes are opened slightly wider than usual.

Breath

Except when otherwise indicated, breathing in Kum Nye dancing always takes place through both nose and mouth, as lightly as possible.

Beginning and ending each session

Before you start your session pause for a moment to take refuge in Kum Nye, validating your inner knowing that Kum Nye is beneficial, and trusting that whatever comes up in your experience will transform as you continue the practice; put your energy and mind into the form.

At the end of a gesture, or when your session is coming to a close and you sit down, be in stillness without 'holding' still ... be ready to dance! As a closing gesture you interlock the fingers of one hand with the fingers of the other and place the back of one hand on the center of the forehead; then reverse the position of the fingers and place the back of the other hand on the same spot. As your hands release, they make a grand opening gesture that ends with briefly placing the hands on the knees with the palms facing up. This closing gesture seals the experience and provides the opportunity to dedicate any merit derived from your session to a person, a group of people, a situation, or to all sentient beings.

Engage with the practices in this book in your own way, and let each gesture inform you about the treasures of your body and mind. It is our hope that as you explore the book, you will discover that each gesture is itself a Kum Nye dance, an encouragement to dance in space, with space. The body and mind are dancing, your embodiment is dancing in space; and space itself is dancing. The expression of joy, is your dancing.

Are you ready to dance?

ARNAUD MAITLAND

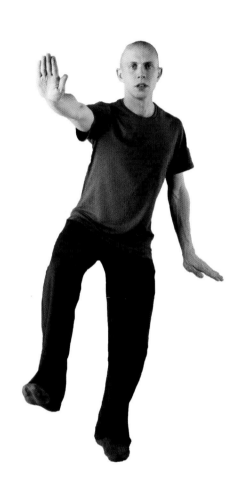

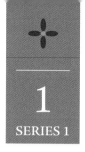

Sense the stillness of the physical body. There is no need to 'hold' still. Stillness will come as longstanding tensions within the body are loosened up and smoothed out, and the oscillations of emotions subside. When the stillness grows more settled, it is possible to dance.

1

Lie on your back, arms alongside the body with the palms flat on the floor. The toes point toward the face. At first, close your eyes gently. Sense the weight of the physical body. Within the heavy body is a lighter body. Slowly open your eyes wide.

2

As you pull up the right knee, interlace the fingers and clasp them around the kneecap. Lift your head and move the forehead toward the knee, while pushing the lower back down. The toes remain flexed. This is more than a stretching exercise; the posture intends to integrate the energy fields of the lower and upper body, enabling them to communicate. Hold the posture.

3

Reverse the posture. Raise the left knee, while stretching the right leg and flexing the feet. Place the interlaced fingers around the left kneecap and bring up your forehead. Go into the stretch, while making the pose increasingly compact.

Repeat each side three times before bringing in rhythm, taking four counts to get into the posture, four counts to hold the posture and four counts to transition into the reverse pose.

Afterward, lie on your right side before coming up to sitting position. Now there is nothing to do but to remain in stillness, without 'holding.'

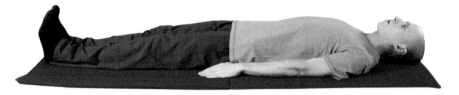

1

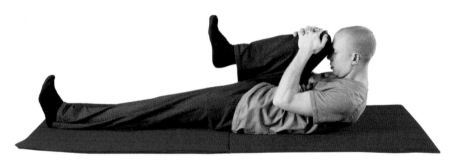

2

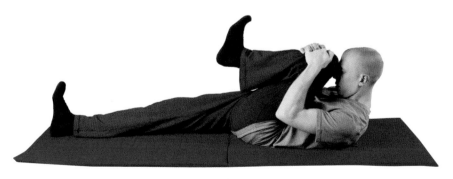

3

As we practice, it is helpful to cultivate a curious, adventurous spirit. Each exercises is a tool for exploration, and the territory is truly new to us. We can think of these exercises as gestures natural and spontaneous expressions of feeling. Organic and inevitable, each gesture is a unique taking place in its own time, and in its own way. It cannot be repeated, for its beauty and appropriateness are in tune with this precise moment, and this precise place in space.

1

Lie on your back, the arms alongside the body. Introduce the mind to the body. The eyes are open wide. Pull up the right knee as high as possible and, while both shoulders remain on the floor, cross the leg over the left hip and twist. Both feet are flexed. The left hand grips the right thigh just above the knee. The right arm remains on the floor at shoulder height, stretching, with the cupped palm up.

2

Return to the center and briefly pause before reversing the movement. This time, the left knee is pulled up high and reaches over the right hip. The right hand supports the thigh. The feet are flexed, and the left arm stretches sideways at shoulder height, with the palm up and the hand slightly cupped.

Become familiar with moving from side to side until a single movement emerges, continuous, as both arms and legs perform in unison.

Repeat three times; then add rhythm.

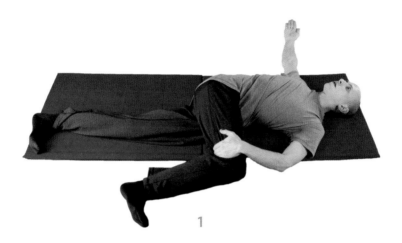

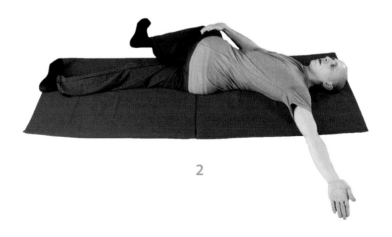

1

2

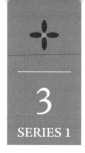

We find that knowledge is not a picture or an idea we keep in our heads—not an overview taken by the mind of the body. The body itself is aware, expressing knowledge.

1

Lie on your back and draw the knees up to the chest. With the hands hold the knees below the kneecaps. The feet are flexed. Make the posture as compact as possible, pushing down on the lower back and lifting the bottom off the floor. Roll to the right side while maintaining this compact position. Briefly hold.

2

Roll back to the center and on to the left side. Briefly hold. Continue going back and forth, side to side, at least ten times before moving on to the next pose. From one point of view it seems as if you are massaging your back. Seen another way, this action is tuning and tending subtle energy. Return to the center and release the posture.

3

Place the feet on the floor and bend the knees at a 45-degree angle. Now, place the left ankle on the right thigh, with the toes flexed. The right hand supports the base of the skull, while the left hand pushes the left thigh down.

Allow the senses to open wide, enabling inner and outer to communicate freely. Sense the way this communication is powered by lower body energy. When you are ready, reverse the position.

At first you may feel differences between the left and right sides, but as you keep alternating from side to side, any differences melt away.

Repeat at least three times before bringing in rhythm.

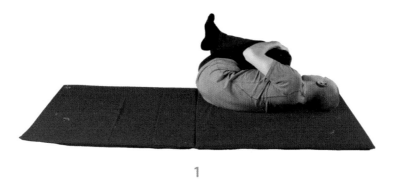

1

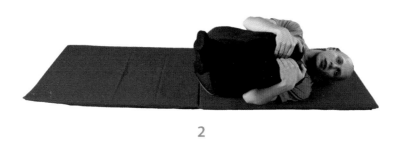

2

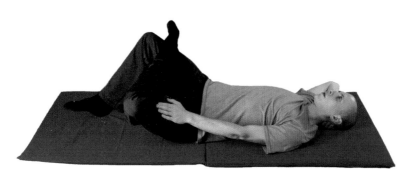

3

4

SERIES 1

Breathing helps you to recognize your intimate connection with the world around you. The air you breathe is not just going in and out of your lungs but unites with and revitalizes the body. Affecting the spirit and mind, the energy of breath plays many roles within the body; it coordinates the relationships of your embodiment.

1

Lie on your back; pull up the knees and keep with the feet on the floor, hip-width apart. The hands are flat on the floor. Feel the texture of the floor or the mat beneath the fingertips. How is your breathing? Is it shallow, hard, anxious, or tense? Let the breath suggest the best way to turn around these feelings.

2

The left hand grips the left hamstring with fingers pointing inwards and the thumb on the outside of the thigh. Stretch the right leg up as much as possible while keeping it straight. The right hand clasps the inside of the knee. The toes of the right foot are flexed. In the transition from pose 1 to 2, did your eyes go blank? Keep them open and actively engaged.

3

Reverse the position as part of one continuous experience. At first, you may feel a difference between the right and the left sides. But over time, the energies flow into each other and each side embodies the qualities of the other side as well.

In the end, return to the starting position and lie on your back with the knees up and the feet flat on the floor. Can you sense the power of the breath moving through the body and coordinating all kinds of relationships?

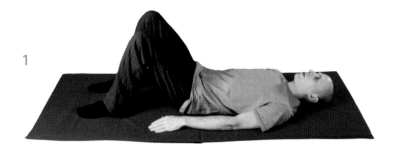

1

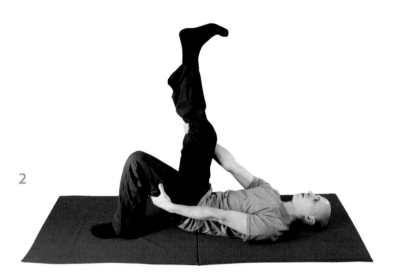

2

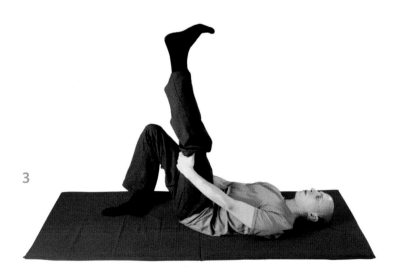

3

5

SERIES 1

Experience shows us that the body can improve its flexibility; we can contact this kind of flexibility directly within feeling. The flexibility of the body, flexibility of feeling, and flexibility of perception are all connected. Gradually, we begin to develop even deeper flexibility; the 'I' itself begins to soften up.

1

Lie on your back with your arms sideways, the palms facing down. The feet are flexed throughout.

2

Pull up the knees into a 45-degree angle, with your feet flat on the floor.

3

Lift the left leg up as high as you can. Push a little, at the same time relaxing into the pose. This pose is not in search of any goal; rather, it is a way to manifest fresh interactions between inner and outer and foster increased mental flexibility.

4

Reverse the pose, lifting the right leg. The left leg remains at a 45-degree angle. During these poses you may at first perceive a difference between the left and right sides, but through repetition the differences vanish.

5

Raise both legs and remain in this position, completing the flexing of body and mind that these postures invite and express. After holding this position return both legs to the ground, back into pose 1.

Repeat at least three times before bringing in rhythm.

∴

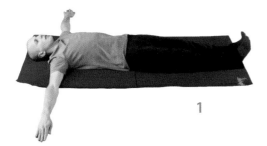

1

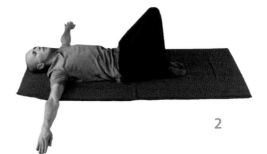

2

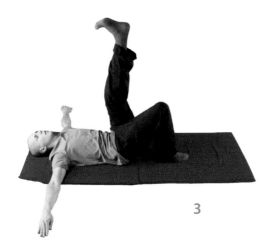

3

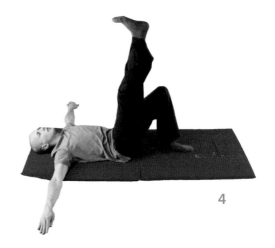

4

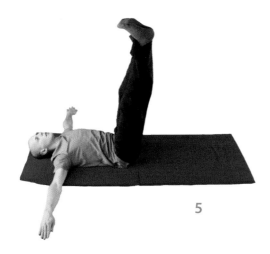

5

Kum Nye works with real-world manifestations and expressions, softening them and easing them toward smoothness. It does not reject the world presented to us by our senses. Instead, Kum Nye massages these structures, slowly opening them up, expanding the range of motion available. Tensions and blockages gradually change. With practice, qualities of experience that seem like hard realities become more malleable.

1

Sit on both sit bones with the back straight. Pull up the knees and place the hands just below the kneecaps. Hold your breath in the navel area and raise the pelvic floor.

2

Holding onto the knees, roll backwards until the lower half of the body is off the floor, resting on the shoulders and the head. Release the breath. Repeat three or nine times. Now you are ready to move in any direction.

3

Return to the sitting position. Place the hands just below the kneecaps and spread the knees to the sides; the soles of the feet are touching. Emphasize the exhalation.

4

Close the knees and wrap the arms around them, holding the upper arms. The head moves forward and down between the knees. The feet are flat on the floor. Emphasize the exhalation.

5

The upper body and arms return to the sitting position. The crossed arms rise all the way over the head. Push the chest forward and up, while stretching the elbows outward and back. Emphasize the inhalation.

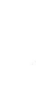

1

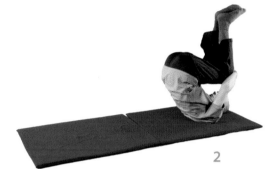

2

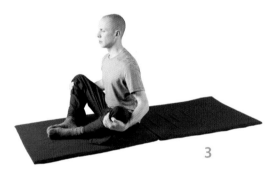

3

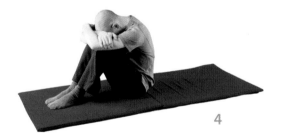

4

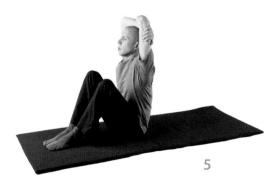

5

Sense impressions are subject to a regime that has been personally and culturally determined over the years. Sensations are immediately connected to images held within conscious awareness and unconscious memory; these connections strengthen each other over time, directing and restricting your experience and understanding. Without noticing, you may be trapped in subtle ways by your mental regime.

1

Sit on your left buttock and place the hands on the floor in front of you; pull up the knees, so the left ankle is resting against the heel of the right foot. There is no need to control this posture. You are not holding on to anything, and nothing is holding onto you. In spite of the awkward position, bathe in stillness–yet be always ready to move.

2

Stretch the right leg and raise it with the toes pointing up and backward. Keeping the right arm straight, firmly grip the lower leg. Remember, you are not controlling anything and nothing is controlling you.

Repeat 1 and 2 three times before moving on to the other side; again, repeat three times before adding rhythm. Hold each position for the same amount of time. Open the eyes wide, embracing space. Focus on sounds; let them come and go without interpretations or definitions. Sound is passing through space, coming from stillness, returning to stillness, in a subtle movement. When unmarked by interpretations, sound is free.

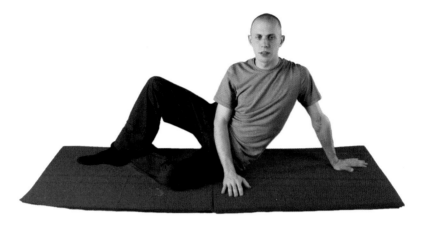

1

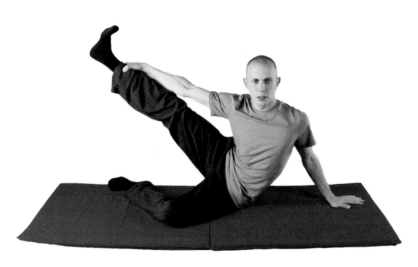

2

Beyond our habitual identifications, as we practice, we may discover that there is really no one in control, only awareness radiating in all directions.

1

Lie on your back, bend the knees and place the feet flat on the floor, a comfortable distance apart. Fold the arms in front of your chest, elbows up, and place the hands just below elbows.

2

From the buttocks on up, raise the upper body at a 45-degree angle. Hold the posture without doubt, worry, or interpretations: remain quietly in present awareness.

3

Twist the torso to the left, opening up the entire left side of your experience. Each step is an invitation to present vivid awareness, new and fresh.

4

Return to the center, briefly pause here and then continue to the right, opening and acknowledging the right side of your experience. Return to the center, lie down and start again, moving in a continuous rhythmic motion, at least three times.

1

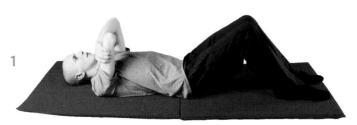

2

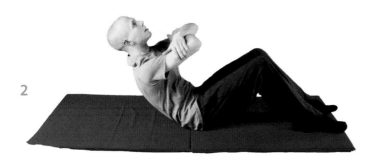

3

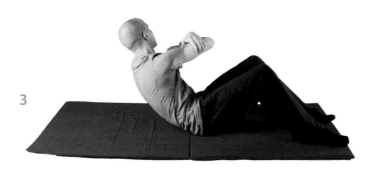

4

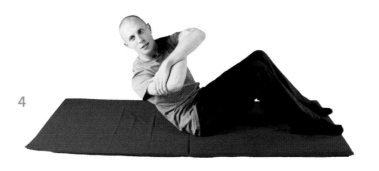

We can become our own natural resource: we can consult within our own experience, and counsel ourselves. When troubles come, we are able to adjust or even substitute the feeling-tones of our choice. By doing this, we find the power to actively engage even unpleasant or unfamiliar experiences.

1

Sit on the floor; pull up the knees and place the feet flat on the floor, touching each other. Each hand grips the leg just below the kneecap. Tilt the head upward and back. Hold the posture.

2

The head returns to the center, briefly pausing before turning to the right. There is no 'you' who is doing it; the head turns on the flow of feeling, expressing flexibility.

The head returns to the center, briefly pausing before turning to the left. During the movement from the right to the left, seeing takes in all of space. There are no gaps in seeing-awareness when you move from one side to the other. The head and the eyes move in unison.

3

Return to the center, briefly pause. Release the arms, interlace the fingers and place them at the back of the head as the torso moves forward and down. The head is in between the knees, the top of the skull pointing straight ahead. The hands slightly press against the back of the head. The elbows are stretching sideways and up.

4

In one fluid movement the upper body comes back up, while the hands, arms and elbows remain in place. The head and the eyes look up at a 45-degree angle. Push the chest forward and up.

Repeat at least three times, before bringing in rhythm.

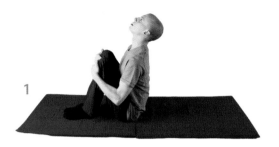

1

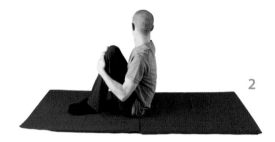

2

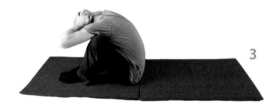

3

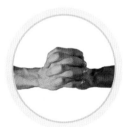

Interlaced

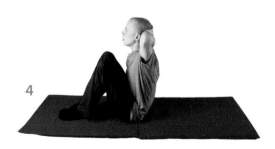

4

10

SERIES 1

As tensions are released, we find that what seemed like obstacles can become our friends. Our bodily experience–our sensations, thoughts and feelings–cradle us as water cradles the swimmer.

1

Sitting up straight, pull up the knees to a 45-degree angle; place the interlaced fingers around the knees and shift your weight onto the left sit bone. The knees move slightly to the left while the torso and the head lean over to the right. The right foot comes off the ground.

2

Return to the center and reverse the posture by shifting onto the right sit bone, and slightly lifting the left foot off the ground. Rock back and forth a few times from one sit bone to the other.

3

Return to the center and sit on both sit bones; separate the knees. Interlace the fingers and place the hands at the base of the skull. The elbows point out as the upper torso comes forward and the head drops down between the knees. The feet are flat on the floor with the insteps touching.

4

In a fluid movement straighten the torso, with the elbows spread apart, opening the armpits. Point the chin upward and look up; apply a slight pressure against the base of the skull.

5

With a grand offering gesture that opens the chest area, spread the arms sideways. The hands are cupped and the palms face upward. Tilt the head back and look up.

Repeat the sequence at least three times before bringing in rhythm.

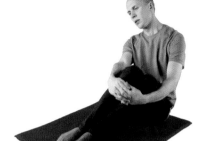

1

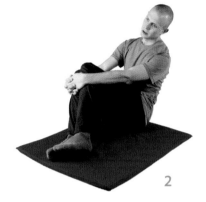

2

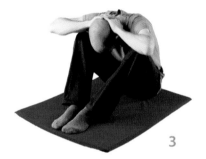

3

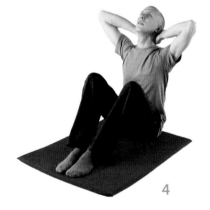

4

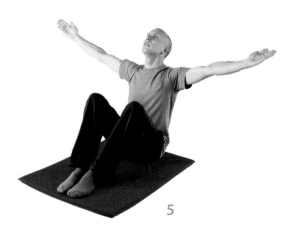

5

11

SERIES 1

Kum Nye restores calmness and clarity and teaches us how to use all the senses, all thoughts, and all facets of our experience. We are able to produce beneficial physical sensations, balanced intellectual concepts, deeper awareness, and healing for the mind. All these qualities are potentially available, but first, we start with the body.

1

Sit upright on your sit bones; pull up the knees into a 45-degree angle and wrap your arms around them.

2

Turn the head and torso all the way to the right, while the arms resist the twist. Pause briefly, and then return to the center. On the way, let your gaze take in all of space so that no gaps in seeing occur.

3

Turn the head from the center to the left.

4

Return the head to the center. In a swift motion lift the arms straight up; the slightly cupped palms face the sky, the fingers point backward, reaching higher and higher.

5

The arms come down sideways until they reach shoulder height, with the cupped palms facing forward.

Repeat at least three times before bringing in rhythm.

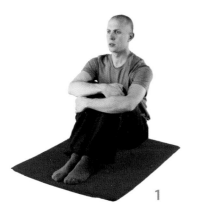

1

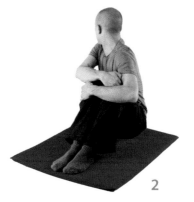

2

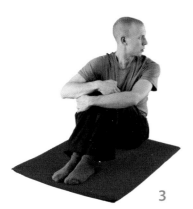

3

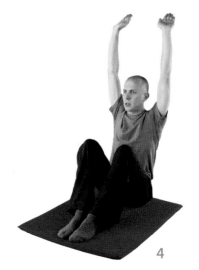

4

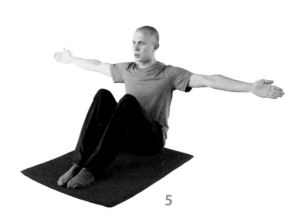

5

12

SERIES 2

Kum Nye practice distills the flavor of bodily experiences into a potent form, in the present moment. This form of practice depends upon flexibility. The subtle interactivity of body and mind is opened up and explored. The power to engage is in the now. We may catch a glimpse of a world we could never imagine.

1

Stand tall with the feet spread wide apart; the toes are pointing outward. Look up at a 45-degree angle, with the eyes wide open.

2

This is the critical part in this set of gestures. Bend the knees to about a 90-degree angle; no further. Place the hands above the knees, thumbs pointing inward. In this position move up and down a few times, until you touch what may feel like the most energizing posture. Settle in and remain there. Look up. Eventually this position will grow on you; it provides the ideal energy for the take-off in any Kum Nye dancing series.

3

Straighten the legs and let the hands slide up. Seeing-awareness remains broad and deep.

Repeat the up-and-down motion three times with rhythmic control.

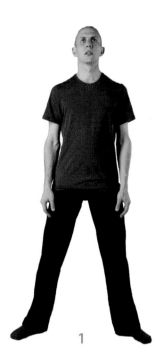

1

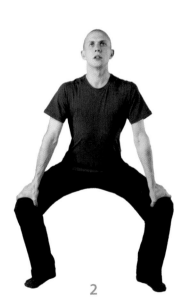

2

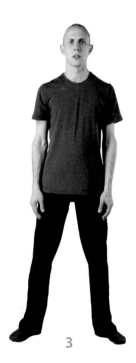

3

We may be unwitting contributors to our tension. Our movements, our attitudes—our very attempts to relax—can tighten up our bodies. As soon as this tension is created, we lose access to the healing qualities of breath energy; this energy begins to stick here and there, locking up in tight corners inside us. When we loosen up, let go of our instructions, and spontaneously embrace our experience, gradually our self-confidence grows. We may not need to fix ourselves after all; perhaps what we really need is to un-fix ourselves. We learned how to be worried, how to be upset; now it is time to un-learn, to wipe the slate clean.

1

In a standing position place the feet at a comfortable distance apart; bend over and place the hands on the floor in front of you, the fingers pointing forward. Straighten the legs as much as possible, while the feet remain flat on the ground. Drop the head in between the arms. Emphasize exhaling.

2

Bend the knees, balancing on the balls of the feet. Lower the buttocks to just above the calves. Raise the head to a horizontal position; the top of the head is pointing forward.

Repeat at least three times, alternating between 1 and 2. Then introduce rhythm for a series of three, nine, or twenty-five times.

Usually this is one of the first postures in a series of movements.

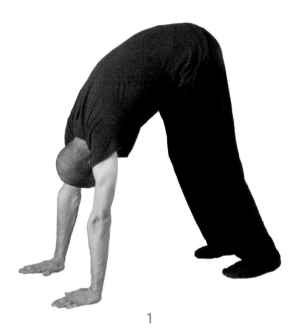

1

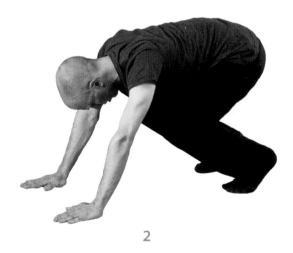

2

Energy travels in waves. The many characters of thoughts, feelings, and physical experiences are in their own fashion waves. When you truly begin to understand this, you need not fear that power. Consider all your experiences as expressions of energy and the movements and gestures you make as waves and ripples. As the breath rises and falls, you can fearlessly experience its many expressions, recognizing for yourself that even obstacles are just waves—fundamental openness, appearing for a brief moment in a certain shape and form.

1

Stand tall and as always, introduce the mind to the body. The arms are relaxed at the sides. Notice if your inner experience of thinking and feeling is moving in waves. Deeply touch the subtle motion underlying all experience.

2

Break up the patterns and energetic structures by bending forward. The head and the arms hang down while the back remains horizontal. Sense the waves of the breath; sense energy traveling in waves.

3

Bend the knees and place the hands on the upper thighs with the thumbs pointing inward and the fingers on the outside. Let the breath rise and fall. Remain in fundamental openness. Straighten the body, releasing the arms, and come back up.

After three repeats, bring in rhythm so that each of the movements has its own character and mixture of sensations.

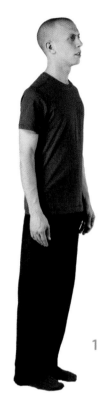

1

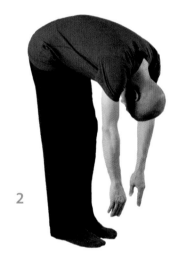

2

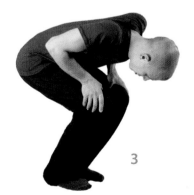

3

15

SERIES 2

Kum Nye practice is designed to penetrate the roots of experience. A new openness arises, beyond the framework of habits, enabling us to leave the corral we have created for ourselves.

1

From a standing position, raise the arms to shoulder height, palms facing down. Bend the knees and lower the pelvis, as if you were to sit down, but not below knee level. The gaze is directed slightly below the horizon.

2

While straightening the legs in this position, in one movement the torso comes to a horizontal position; the arms go down and the fingers point toward the ground. The top of the head points forward.

3

In a swinging motion the upper body and the arms come up, the palms facing forward and the fingers pointing toward the sky. The armpits are opening. The gaze is directed slightly above the horizon, taking in all of space.

Repeat three times, in a continuous movement; then bring in rhythm.

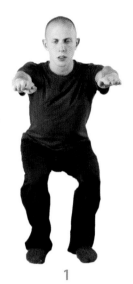

1

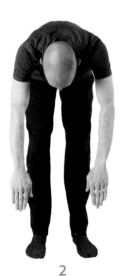

2

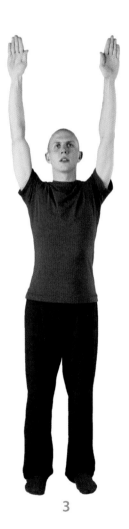

3

Is it possible that all sensations communicate at bottom? Perhaps all of them, without exception, have the power to conduct us beyond ourselves to the same place-less place— the open field.

1

In a standing position, place the feet a comfortable distance apart; throughout the posture the body weight is equally divided over both feet. Interlock the fingers and place them at the base of the skull; arch to the right, stretching and opening the left armpit. The elbows point up and slightly back. Hold the posture.

2

Return to the center; briefly pause before moving on to the opposite side. Open the right armpit. Hold the posture.

3

Return to the center. Slightly bend the knees, as the upper torso moves forward to a horizontal position. The elbows are pointing to the sides. Do not drop the head; the top of the head points forward. Apply pressure to the base of the skull.

4

In one fluid movement, straighten the legs and swing the upper body all the way up; wide open eyes invite new experiences to enter.

When you are ready, bring in rhythm.

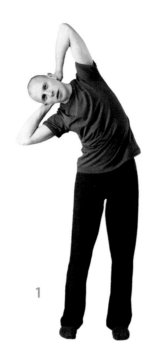

1

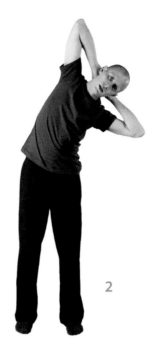

2

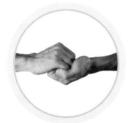

Interlocked

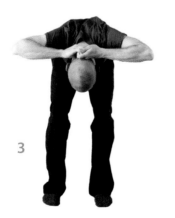

3

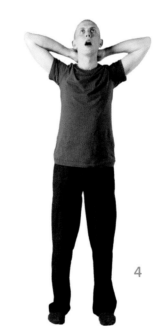

4

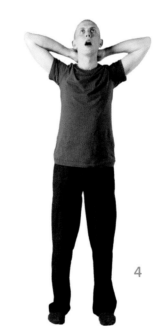

17

SERIES 2

The soil of the mind is extraordinarily fertile. It will accept and foster a startling range of experiences, joyful and terrible. But once we have really penetrated the structure of our sense-experience, really seen our own regimented thinking at work, really experienced our feelings as ripples expanding in openness, the chain that binds our inward responses to our outward circumstances is broken. Nothing obligates us to suffer.

1

In a standing position, with the arms at the sides, place the feet hip-width apart. The eyes penetrate the space ahead. Fully engage the body, especially the legs and the feet. Lift the right knee up high with the foot flexed, the toes pointing upward.

2

Rather rapidly, reverse the posture; the right leg comes down as the left knee comes up. Alternate legs, stomping vigorously as your feet touch the ground.

3

Keeping your body upright, bend at the knees, lowering the buttocks toward the ground as if to sit down. The back remains straight throughout. Continue to move your legs up and down, pounding the heels into the ground.

4

Go down as deeply as you can. Increase the speed of the movements until the motion of up and down and the stomping of the ground become irregular and chaotic.

Stop suddenly, stand up straight and be still. Now, let yourself feel.

Repeat at least three times, each time lifting the knees higher and stamping the feet more vigorously.

∴

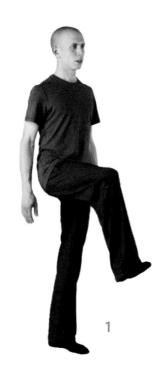

1

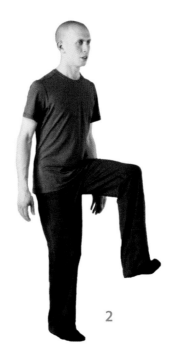

2

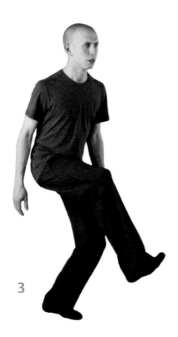

3

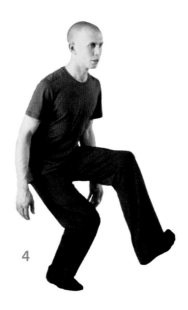

4

18

SERIES 2

Are we truly living in the present tense? As we recognize that we are not present, the moment of recognition has the power to engage us in the now

1

Stand tall and raise the arms to shoulder height. Bend the arms at the elbows so that they form 90-degree angles. Bend the wrists so that the palms of the hands face toward the sky. The eyes, directed upward at a 45-degree angle, are wide open.

2

Stretch the arms above the head, sensing the connection between the heart and hands as you lift the heart energy to the sky. At the same time, the eyes gaze straight up beyond the outstretched hands. Extend energy and awareness through the palms as you continue to reach towards the sky.

3

Keeping the elbows bent, bring the arms back to shoulder height. As the arms descend, invite the qualities of the sky into the body and senses, receiving and absorbing them.

4

Repeat posture 2. The gaze remains stable, expansive yet penetrative. Experiment with postures 3 and 4 three, nine, or twenty-five times before bringing in rhythm.

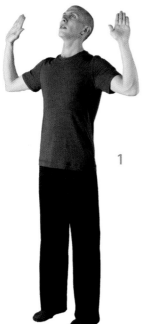

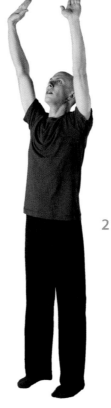

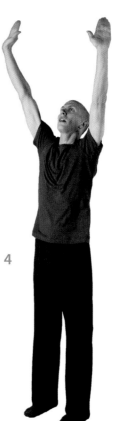

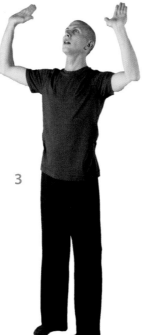

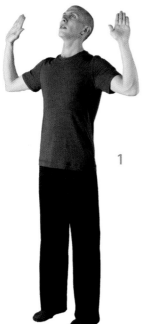

1

2

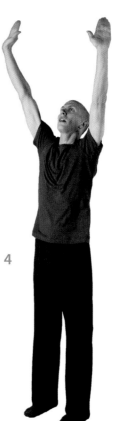

18
SERIES 2

3

4

Beyond the pre-patterned character of experience, beyond all mental activity, there may exist a completely different reality—a total openness. We discover that we have what we need and that we are what we seek: like space, we are already open.

1

Place the legs wide apart and, with the palm of the hand slightly cupped, lift the right arm. The eyes look into space just to the left of the outstretched hand. The left arm is pointing downward, and the palm of the hand is cupped.

2

Reverse the posture so that the left arm reaches up, with the left hand slightly cupped and facing towards the sky. Meanwhile the right arm stretches down with the right palm cupped, facing down. Sky and earth meet within us and their union is expressed through the rhythm of the body. No control, no plans, no waiting for it to be over, but completely expressing the present moment.

Perform each step three or nine times before you bring in rhythm. Experiment with both slowing down and increasing the pace.

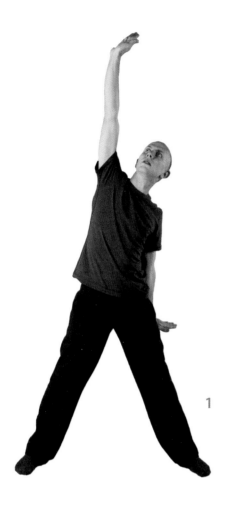

1

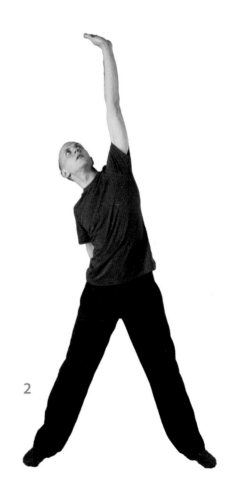

2

There is no need to make 'being in the present' the goal of practice. On the contrary: striving prevents awareness from opening up. Presence can just be, and relaxation comes naturally, further opening the present moment, ocean-wide.

1

Stand straight, with the arms relaxed at your sides and the legs spread wide apart, the toes pointing outward. Emphasize gentle exhalations; notice the interactions of sensations and feelings.

2

Place the left hand above the left knee with the thumb pointing in and the fingers pointing out, in a vigorous hold. Raise the right arm, arching it overhead to the left, with the cupped palm facing forward. The arm and hand form a horizontal line. The posture penetrates space with the right arm, while at the same time loosening up lower body energies. New contacts and new relationships may emerge.

3

Reverse the posture. The grip and the reaching are constantly intensifying.

Repeat three times before bringing in rhythm.

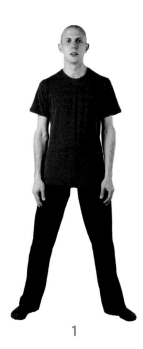

1

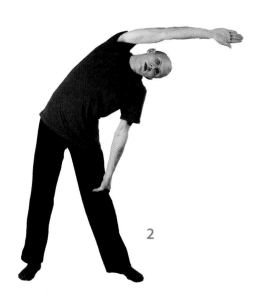

2

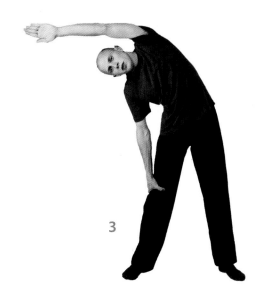

3

21

SERIES 2

As we learn to deepen relaxation, the body gets more juice; it is nourished by joy, and set free from distraction. Tensions melt away; we settle into calmness, not separate and alone, but part of a whole, at one with our environment. Releasing tension, we reach a moment of exquisite balance, a resting point of ease.

1

Stand straight and lift the arms in front of you to shoulder height, with the cupped palms of the hands facing down. Draw in the left arm, pointing the left elbow backward; both arms are aligned. The left hand remains close to the chest, with the palm down. The right arm continues to reach forward. Gather all energies in preparation for the next pose.

2

Reverse the position, keeping the arms on the same plane. Push the left arm forward, as if cutting through space and hitting a target. Simultaneously draw in the right arm, as if pulling a bow and arrow. The extended arm is aligned with the upper arm that is drawn back; the right hand is held close to the chest, the cupped palm facing down. Briefly hold the posture, making it tight and sharp. Throughout, the eyes remain strongly directed forward, the gaze aimed just above the extended hand.

Alternate at least ten times before bringing in rhythm. Experiment with speeding up, increasing the swiftness of the movement, clearing all confusion and uncertainties.

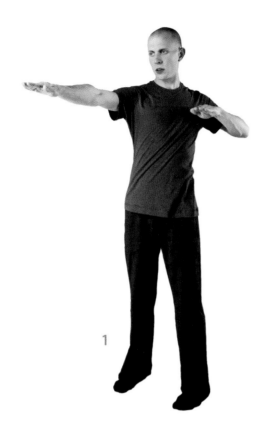

1

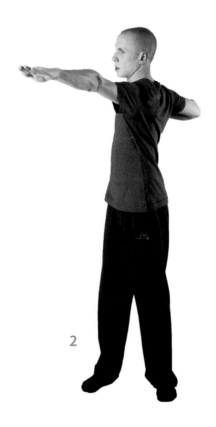

2

With Kum Nye, we begin to discover the soothing qualities in the body experience and learn to openly contact the varied flavors of our sense of feeling. In making these contacts, as we soften the intensity of our attachments, more new flavors of feeling will emerge. When the bonds to our orientation are loosened up, new energies are set free; instead of being tethered to subject and object, awareness becomes independent.

1

Sit upright on both sit-bones; the knees are pulled up with the feet flat on the floor. The hands are on the floor beside you, with the palms up. Emphasize the exhalation.

2

Interlace the fingers, and place them at the base of the skull. Bend the torso forward, spread the knees and move the head forward and down. The palms of the hands apply light pressure against the back of the head. If you are flexible, the top of the head points forward. The elbows are spread apart, the armpits are open. Take time to surrender to the posture, not by 'holding', but by resting in it, as if you might stay like this, effortlessly, for a long time. Make contact with any new flavors within experience.

3

Come upright in one fluid motion. With the hands still behind the head, spread the elbows apart, tilt the head back, open the mouth wide in a circle and look up. Remain like this in stillness for a while. After releasing the posture return to sitting in stillness, manifesting a free, independent awareness.

Repeat the movement three times before bringing in rhythm. Experiment with increasing the speed of the flow, or slowing down.

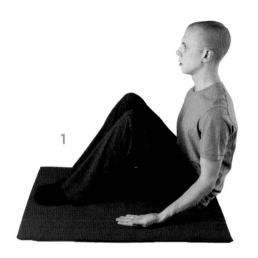

1

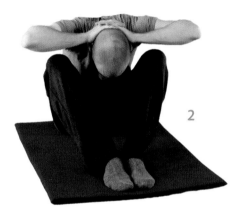

2

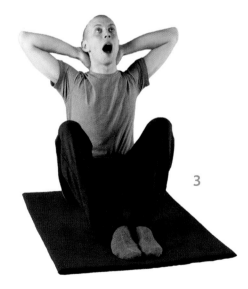

3

It is important to develop knowledge of your own body. Each human body has its own needs, different from others, with different habits and different ways of expressing itself. Working closely with yourself, you can find the approach that suits your mind and energy best. Exploring the body, we learn that all experience is an expression of a fundamental unity.

1

Sit up straight and pull up the knees, wrapping the arms around them. Look straight ahead, penetrating the depths of open space. You are not holding on to anything, and nothing is holding on to you. There is no grasping, no aversion; no sinking, no elation. This is neutral openness.

2

Bring the chin forward, placing it between the knees. The eyes keep looking straight ahead, at a level just below the horizon.

Sitting in these two postures, you seem not to be doing anything. Yet at a subtle level, the flexibility of the body is manifesting itself in different shapes and forms.

The postures are expressions of energy, displaying different states of mind and being.

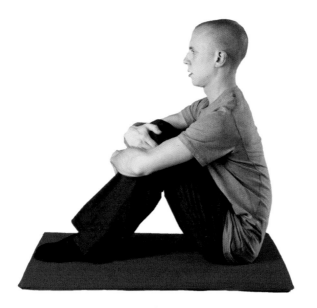

1

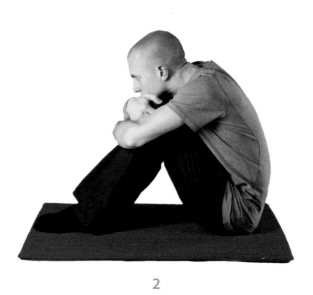

2

Without controlling the breath, we can allow it to move through us, relaxing the belly, the heart, and the throat. Breath moves smoothly, filling and nourishing each cell as we inhale, tapering off almost imperceptibly as we exhale. Although they can seem sharp and stark, our sense-experiences too are moving, changing, filling us through and through and gradually dispersing.

1

Lie on your back with the arms alongside the body, the palms flat on the floor. Pull up the knees while keeping the feet on the floor, slightly spread apart. Without controlling the breath, allow it to move through the body while relaxing the belly, the heart, and the throat.

2

Place the right foot on the left knee and the right hand on the right knee. Raise the bottom, while keeping the torso on the floor.

3

The bottom is lowered to the floor, as the right leg crosses over the left thigh. The right foot and toes are flexed.

4

Pull up the left knee and clasp your hands around it. As the knees are drawn to the chest, the bottom comes off the floor. Grip firmly and make the posture compact, without dropping the left leg to the center. The toes are flexed. Notice that sense experiences may seem sharp and stark at first, but like the breath, they too are moving, changing, and gradually dispersing. Reverse the position.

Repeat at least three times, without controlling the breath. When you are ready, bring in rhythm.

1

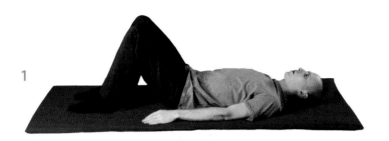

2

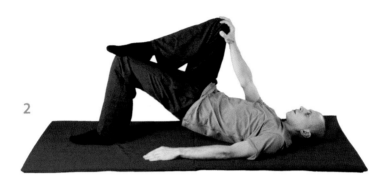

3

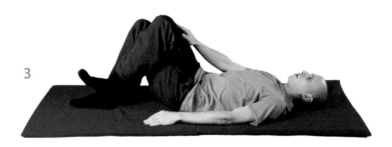

4

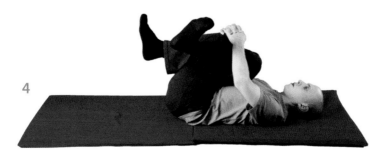

We can cultivate and protect our inner resources, so they never run dry. When those resources are fully developed there is no need to hang on to hope or dogmatically convince ourselves that we chose the right path. We have total confidence, based on the evidence of the senses.

1

Lie on your back with the palms of the hands facing down. Count backwards from 4 to 1, and then bring the left knee up to the chest. Hold it firmly with your left hand just below the kneecap. Then raise the right leg, keeping it as straight as possible. With the right hand, hold the back of the hamstring. Finally, if you can, lift the bottom off the ground, while pushing the lower back down. The feet are flexed throughout.

2

Moving arms and legs at the same time, reverse the position. Transitioning demands the same quality of attention as the posture itself. Keep your bottom off the floor through the transition, if you can.

3

With the hands supporting the hamstrings, straighten both legs while stretching them.

4

Open the legs as wide as possible, while gripping the thighs with the hands.

Throughout the practice, keep your eyes open wide.

Repeat at least three times before bringing in rhythm.

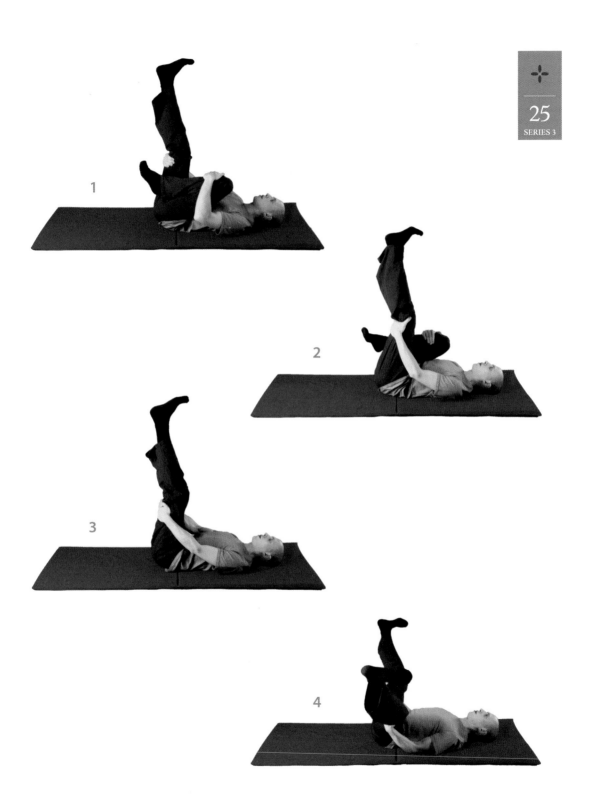

1

2

3

4

Breath is a manifestation of the state of mind and body. It shows how we are feeling. Being preoccupied or anxious can make it hard to breathe, as if the space for the breath is already full, and then creates further anxiety. Breathing practice can teach us how to use the breath to turn this situation around and direct experience to openness. As the breath moves through the body, it refines, extracts, purifies, and alchemizes.

1

Lie on your back. Flex the feet and pull up the right knee. Place the left ankle directly below the right kneecap, interlacing the fingers around the shin. If possible, lift the bottom off the ground, while pressing down the lower back. The eyes are wide open.

2

Straighten the right leg, while moving the hands around to grip the hamstrings. The feet remain flexed throughout. During the transition, the eyes remain open wide, without blinking or going blank.

3

Return to the center and briefly pause before reversing the posture. Pull up the left knee and, while the right ankle crosses over the left kneecap, hold the shin. The movements should be a continuous experience.

4

From this position, stretch the left leg while gripping the left hamstrings.

5

Release the hands; pull up both knees to the chest and place the hands just below the kneecaps.

Repeat three times on each side and then bring in rhythm if you like. When you are finished, before coming up, turn onto the right side with the knees pulled up, resting for a moment.

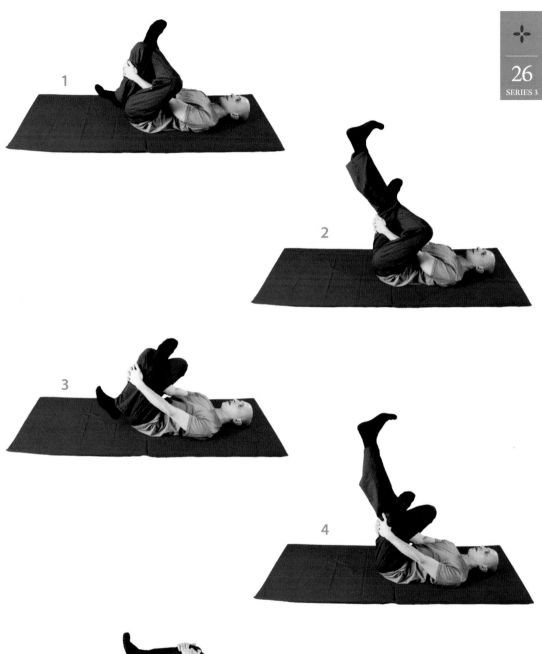

1

2

3

4

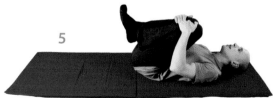

5

Even when we are not actively practicing Kum Nye, we can work in a Kum Nye way with experience, becoming conscious of physical and emotional habits, and allowing our ordinary thoughts, feelings and movements to become our teachers.

1

Lie on your back, legs out straight. The right leg crosses over the left; the feet are flexed, toes pointing toward your face. Place the hands on the stomach and solar plexus: the left hand is pointing to the right, and below it the right hand is pointing to the left. Sense the texture of your clothing against the palms and fingertips. The eyes are wide open and receptive. Introduce breath and mind to the area in the body below the palms of the hands. Welcome sensations, feelings and interactions between them with interested curiosity. Stay alert and engaged as these interactions change and evolve.

2

Reverse the positions of the legs and the hands. Stay with any evolving internal experiences, intent on getting to know them deeply.

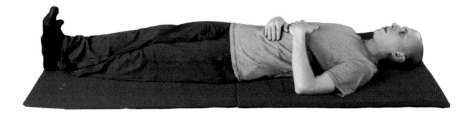

1

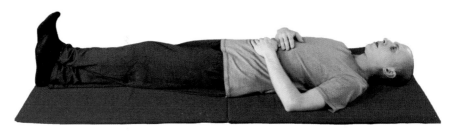

2

Kum Nye breathing practices can lead to profound self-mastery, even altering the body down to the cellular level. Gradually, as breathing expands awareness, ordinary ways of inhabiting the body and experiencing the world begin to change. Through new breathing patterns it may be possible to create different ways of embodying.

1

Lie on your left side with the left arm tucked under the head. Place the palm of the right hand on the floor in front of the solar plexus, the fingers pointing toward the left elbow. The right leg is resting on top of the left leg. Pull up the knees and flex the feet. The eyes are soft and expansive.

2

Sharpen the posture, including the eyes. Raise both legs off the ground and hold, pushing with the right hand. Hold the posture for thirty to sixty seconds and gradually lengthen its duration. Then, lower the legs to the ground. Be still, without 'holding' still, and listen to the breath. How deep does it travel now?

Then reverse the position, making sure that postures 1 and 2 are of equal duration. In the beginning, the experience on the left and right sides may be different. But gradually, through Kum Nye dancing, a unified being moves and explores.

Repeat three times before bringing in rhythm.

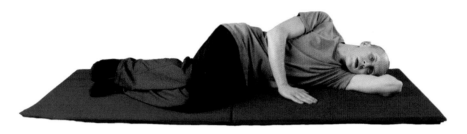

1

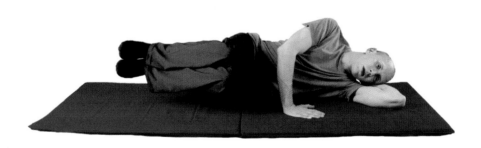

2

Locked away inside the individual lie many positive qualities, including depth of feeling, hidden talents, and intelligence. Kum Nye can help us to discover these qualities, and practice can help them to emerge unobstructed by fear.

1

Lie on your back with the arms alongside the body, the palms of the hands flat on the floor. Sense the body making contact with the earth below. Introduce the mind to the body. Turn onto the left side, keeping the legs straight. The right leg is resting on the left, and the toes are flexed. The eyes are wide open; the gaze is quiet, neutral. Bring the left arm across the upper chest and heart region to the other side; the fingertips touch the ground. As the head moves to the right, the gaze fans from the center to the right, taking in all of space.

2

Reverse the position, shifting onto the right side, again lining up the legs. As the head moves, the eyes follow. At the same time, cross the right arm over the chest and heart region. The left fingers are touching the earth. Hold the posture.

Repeat the movement on both sides three times. Then bring in rhythm for another three repetitions.

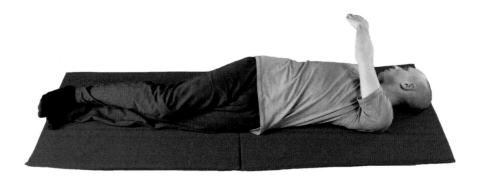

1

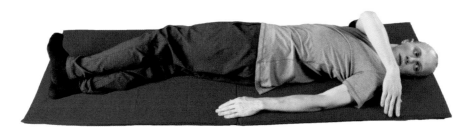

2

30

The body may have limits to its flexibility, but the mind knows no such constraints. Awareness is infinitely flexible; expanding and condensing, embracing and accommodating. As you develop greater flexibility in your senses and responses, breathing can be your teacher. As you take in air, your lungs gently expand. The feeling of air going in, of the lungs opening up, is a direct and nourishing experience of flexibility. The air freely going out as you exhale— that is also flexibility.

1

Sit upright on both sit-bones, with the knees drawn up to the chest. The feet are flat on the floor, with the insteps touching. Place the hands flat on the floor, next to your bottom, with the fingers pointing forward. The arms are straight, causing the shoulders to rise. The chin is slightly tucked in; the eyes look strongly toward a point in infinite space. Settle in the posture without 'holding' it.

2

Wrap the arms around the knees. Raise the chin slightly; the eyes are still looking straight ahead, but the gaze is now softer and more open to the sides.

Repeat expanding and condensing awareness, as described in 1. Can you imagine expanding this feeling of flexibility until you accommodate the universe?

At first, hold the poses for about one minute, but gradually extend the duration of each pose.

∴

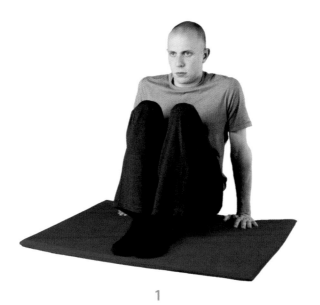

1

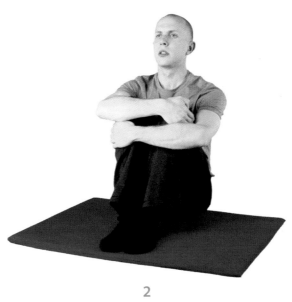

2

Kum Nye is a gradual approach that works with the grain of experience, using our human condition as a sacred vehicle of transformation.

1

In a sitting position lift the arms to shoulder height and, with clenched fists, stretch them out.

2

Keep the back straight throughout the gestures. Bend the elbows, drawing them back, and bring the forearms to the sides, parallel to each other.

3

Twist the upper torso to the right and move the arms to the right and back, keeping them at the same level. The head faces forward.

4

Swing the arms to the opposite side in a sweeping motion.

5

Return to the center with the arms at shoulder height, elbows bent and pointing down. Release the fists and cup the hands, with the fingers pointing up.

6

Swiftly push the accumulated energy upwards, leaving the body empty and clear. The arms are straight above the head and the palms are flat, facing the sky.

7

Lower the arms sideways; bend the elbows at a 45-degree angle and make fists at shoulder level. In a vigorous motion, push the hands forward into position 1.

With each movement the power in the fists, arms and body increases. The motions are swift and almost abrupt.

Repeat at least three times before bringing in rhythm.

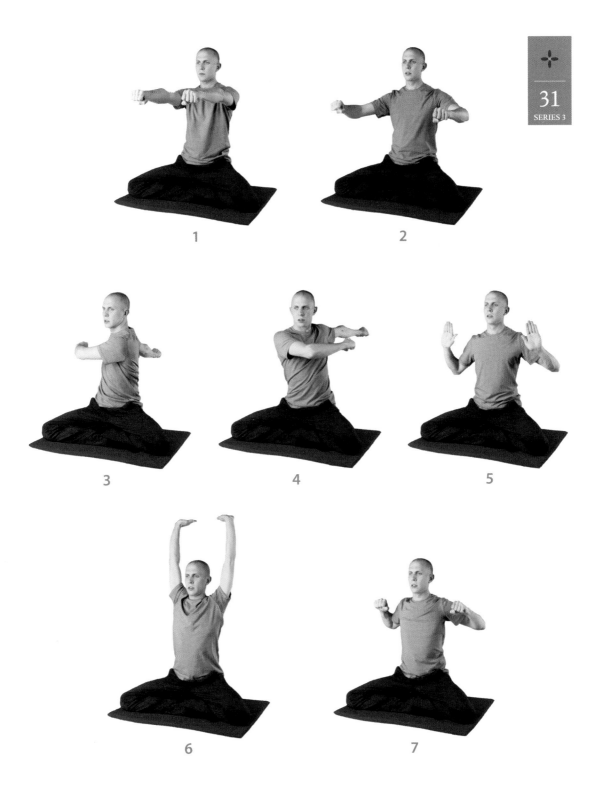

1

2

3

4

5

6

7

Once we have touched the depths of sense-experience, tasted that unchangeable essence, and fully realized our basic openness, the beauty of being pours in on all sides.

1

The energy in the palms of the hands plays a role in exploring inner and outer space. This energy can be awakened and applied. Slightly cup the hands and begin to rub them back and forth.

2

Increase the speed of the rubbing. There is no need to add any mental activity to this rubbing back and forth, like imagining more heat or wondering about the purpose of it all. All there is is the rigorous massaging of the palms, with the body fully engaged.

3

The hands move toward the eyes. As the palms cover the convex shape of the eyes, the fingers cover the forehead. At first, this gesture may simply help cultivate relaxation. Eventually, it will facilitate the communication between the inner world and the outer dimensions of space.

4

After rubbing the hands again in front of the heart, bring them up to the ears, the palms covering the concave shape of the ears. In a similar manner as with the eyes, the energy in the palms connects deeply with the inner world of hearing beyond meaning.

Afterward sit in stillness, without 'holding' still.

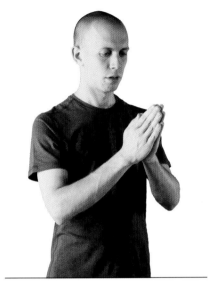

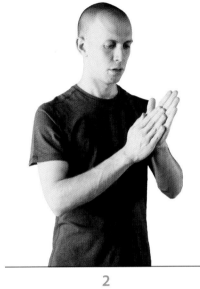

1

2

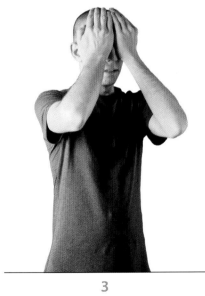

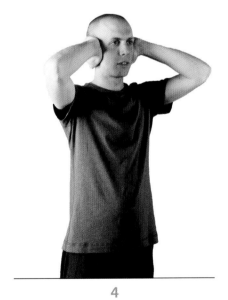

3

4

You are one with the body; this understanding is essential to unlocking the transformative potential of Kum Nye. To enhance this process, treat the body with kindness, for it is not an object you possess; it is intimately yourself.

1

Stand with the feet a comfortable distance apart, the arms relaxed alongside the body and the fingertips touching your clothing, sensing its texture. Slowly and carefully turn the head to the right, opening the left side of the neck. Look far into the distance.

2

Tilt the head slightly backward, but not all the way; the chin is pointing sideways. This posture may unfix tension. Embrace the sensations and feelings, even painful ones.

3

The head slowly continues to roll backwards, bypassing the middle back position until it reaches the opposite tilted position. There is no need to focus on practice or on sensations. Rather, you are embracing the experience, be it tense, painful, or neutral.

4

After coming up straight, the head turns to the left, as close as possible to a 90-degree angle, opening the right side of the neck. Return to the center.

Repeat several times, emphasizing the four positions. When you are ready, bring in rhythm.

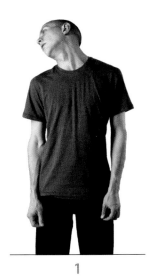

1

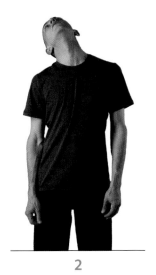

2

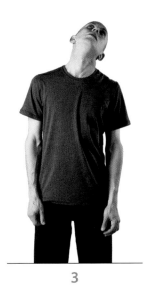

3

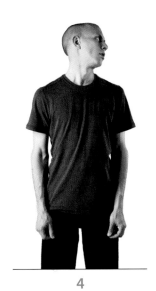

4

When you get more familiar with the internal qualities of your experience, your initial reactions to what is happening begin to change. Eventually even challenging sensations can be encompassed by curious, sensitive, open awareness. Awareness that simultaneously takes good care of you and keeps you safe and free from fear. Without fear, without craving, sensitivity grows finer and awareness expands.

1

Stand with the feet at a comfortable distance apart, the hands firmly gripping the lower arms and holding them close to the body. Pull in the navel and slightly raise the shoulders throughout 1-3. The eyes are soft and gaze down at a 45-degree angle.

2

Slightly increase the overall tension, as the head leans to the left, the ear approaching the left shoulder as much as possible and lengthening the right side of the neck. Like all the other gestures, these movements manifest flexibility, supported by the flow of energy.

3

The head returns to the center and gently moves to the opposite side.

4

Release the arms, navel and shoulders at the same time, while the head drops forward, showing a different kind of flexibility.

Repeat three times.

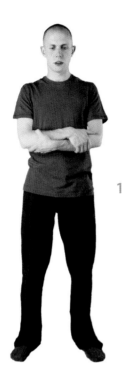

1

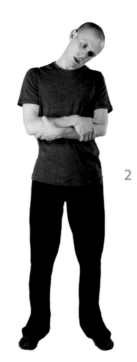

2

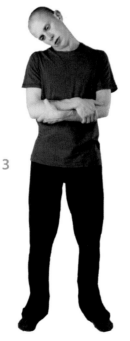

3

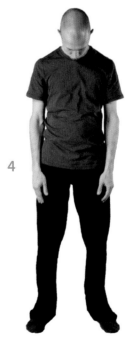

4

35

SERIES 4

For all beings, the senses are mediating experience. Our senses are the part of us that connects with the rest of the world, and each sense has its own specific, characteristic way of engaging and relaying its signals. The senses condition not just how we perceive, but also how we feel and think. While we share certain basic operations and structures, each sense faculty is distinct: no two people see the same thing in precisely the same way.

1

In a standing position, with the feet at a comfortable distance apart, fold the arms and hold them up in front of the chest, gripping the upper arms with the hands. In this set of movements, the eyes play an important role. The eyes are soft and expansive.

2

The upper torso bends to the left; the folded arms and gripping hands follow. Seeing takes on a different angle.

3

Return to the center and bend to the opposite side. The eyes travel into new dimensions.

4

Return to the center and raise the crossed arms over the head and even further backward, opening the armpits. Release the arms, lowering them sideways and begin again with 1.

Repeat three times. When you are ready, bring in rhythm.

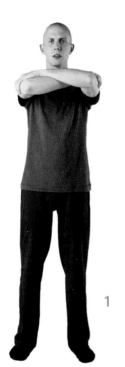

1

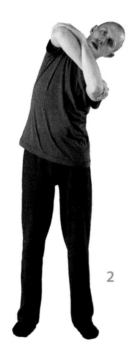

2

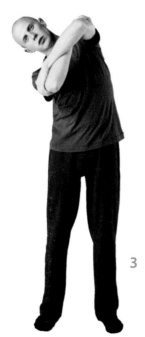

3

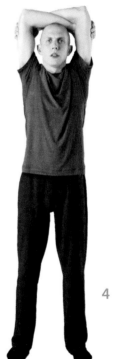

4

36

SERIES 4

Kum Nye is more than an exercise regime; it is a system of embodied knowledge. If practiced deeply and sincerely, it can lead to a transformation of the human condition. Tibetan masters transmitted knowledge beyond concepts, using the vehicle of human embodiment. Kum Nye is part of this lineage.

1

The hands grasp the lower arms in front of the chest. The grip is firm and secure. The gaze is stable, unmoving. The body is loose and flexible, prepared to move in any direction.

2

While the lower body remains stationary, the upper torso twists to the right; head and eyes follow the movement of the torso. It is easy to become preoccupied with performing the movements perfectly—instead, allow the head to turn as if by itself. Body, mind, and seeing move in unison.

3

The upper body, head, and eyes move through the center to the other side.

Move with the flow of feeling, rather than from will power. Let the flow of feeling support the movements and direct the openings. Explore new directions with seeing as a two-way channel, unifying outward and inward in open seeing.

Repeat at least three times before bringing in rhythm.

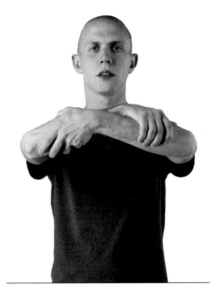

1

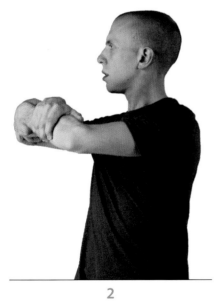

2

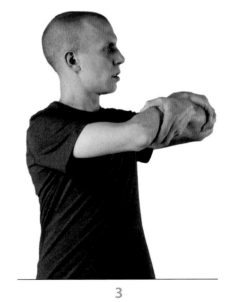

3

Kum Nye shows that we need not make enemies with any part of experience. The qualities of experience all emerge from constant relation and interaction with our inner and outer environments. An intricate dance is taking place within us; an animated conversation is being held. Consciousness trained by Kum Nye practice can engage directly with experience and foster positive interactions. Kum Nye is the art of making friends with all experience.

1

In a standing position, place the feet at a comfortable distance apart. With curious interest, make contact with internal and external experiences. These are always changing and are intensified by the movements and postures.

The arms move forward to shoulder height, with the palms of the hands facing down.

2

Bend the knees and move the upper body down to a horizontal position; the arms and hands reach straight ahead, the cupped palms facing down. Keep reaching and stretching. The top of the head points forward. Acknowledge each new experience, developing awareness of the ongoing conversations that emerge from the interaction with your inner and outer environments. Hold the posture.

3

In one fluid movement straighten the legs and swing the upper body and arms all the way up. Look beyond the outstretched arms, deep into the sky. Hold the posture, making friends with experience.

Repeat three times. When you are ready, bring in rhythm.

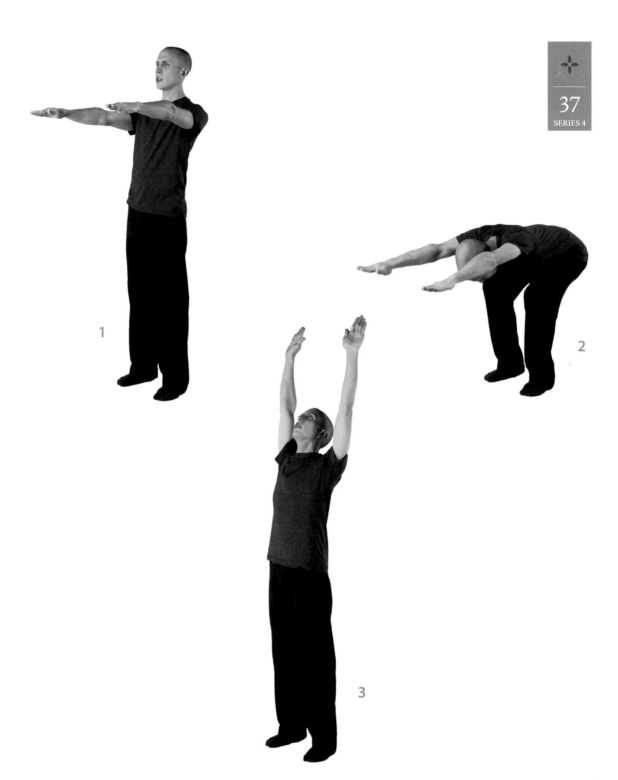

1

2

3

38

SERIES 4

The postures and practices in this book are invigorating rather than soothing, designed to energize the body and to wake up consciousness.

1

In a standing position place your feet widely apart, toes pointing out, not sideways. Bend the torso forward from the waist into a horizontal position. Place the hands on the legs above the knees, with the thumbs pointing inward. The back remains flat and the arms straight. The breath is light, almost unnoticeable.

2

While the left leg remains straight, the right knee begins to bend over the right foot. Next, shift your weight to the right. Press down with the right hand while the right shoulder comes forward. Push the buttocks sideways and down. The back and the arms remain straight. The gaze is stable. Hold the posture.

3

In one sweeping motion, shift your weight to the left leg, pressing down with the left arm and moving the left shoulder forward. At the same time the right leg straightens out, and the buttocks go down and out.

At first there may be a difference in energy or feeling level between the left and right sides, but any differences will gradually disappear.

Repeat three or nine times and feel how the shifting back and forth becomes a light body twist from side to side. Finally, bring in rhythm.

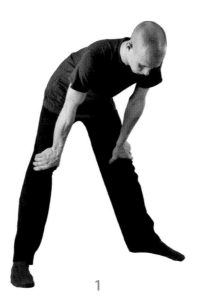

1

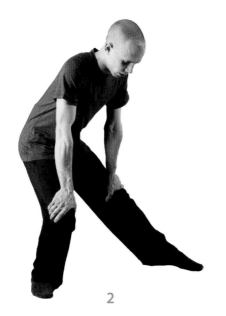

2

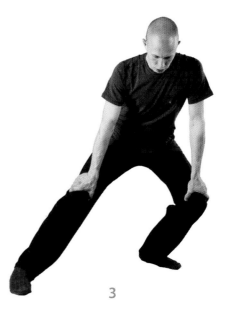

3

The qualities of our experience are emerging from constant relationships with one another and with space; an intricate dance is taking place within us, an animated conversation with many participants is being held. Awareness itself is not separate from these interactions, but part of the conversation, emerging from and contributing to its endless unfolding. Consciousness trained by Kum Nye practice can engage directly with regimes of thoughts, senses, and emotions, fostering positive interactions.

1

Standing tall, place the feet wider apart than usual. Raise the arms in front of you until they are at shoulder height, with the cupped hands facing down; stretch the arms, hands and fingertips forward while maintaining a straight back.

2

Simultaneously the arms, hands, and head move to the right, synchronized with one another.

3

Devote yourself to becoming fluid in moving from side to side. The act of moving the arms is as important as the final posture. Shift without the notion of going from one place to another; be fully engaged in moving.

Repeat three times before adding rhythm, each time increasing the experience of the present.

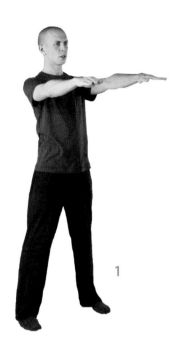

1

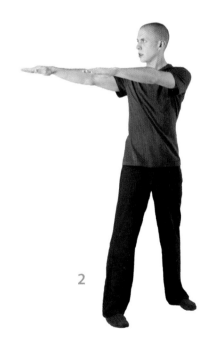

2

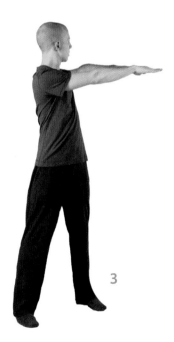

3

40

SERIES 4

The gestures of Kum Nye set clear goals, lay out methods to follow, and offer gentle ways to focus energy and attention. If they are practiced with care, they can at the very least improve our well-being, enriching the soil of our experiences, strengthening our trust in our senses, and allowing us to access a deeper sense of our own aliveness.

1

Stretch your arms in front of you at shoulder height, the cupped palms almost touching. The eyes are wide open. Briefly hold this posture.

2

Begin to widen the space between the palms to shoulder-width, with the cupped hands held parallel. Move the hands back and forth, together and apart, gradually increasing speed until the hands move as fast as possible. Still the hands never touch, nor do they extend beyond shoulder-width. Continue for a few moments; then pause with the hands at heart level, the palms almost touching.

3

Now the vertical movements begin. As the left arm moves up, the right arm moves down.

4

Reach up and down as far as possible, cutting sharply through space. The lower hand reaches slightly behind the leg.

Bring the movements to a close in front of the chest as in posture 1.

Repeat three or nine times. Once the steps and movements are fluid, give attention to rhythm and timing.

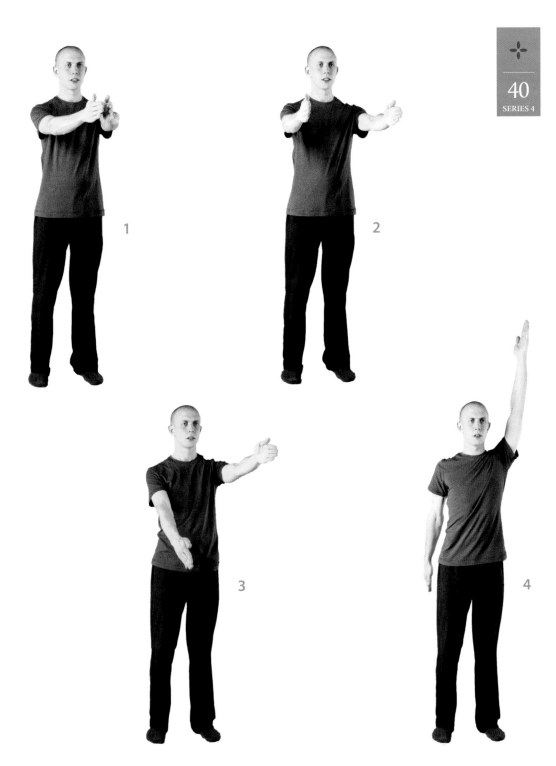

1

2

3

4

The first step in Kum Nye dancing is to learn how to get seated in experience. We can think of Kum Nye development as a gradual settling down into this seat. At first, we may receive only little tastes of this quality, but over time as we continue to practice, we encounter a calmness that does not disperse easily when thoughts and sensations come. It becomes possible to remain in calmness, to keep our seat. Senses, experiences, thoughts and feelings come and go, but calmness remains, allowing us to make contact with the subtle, balanced, sustaining depths of practice.

1

In a standing position, place your feet at hip width. The arms move up sideways to shoulder height, with the cupped palms of the hands facing down. Make contact with the entire body. Equally divide the weight of the body over the two feet throughout the postures.

2

While the hips remain in place, the left arm moves forward and the right arm backward; the head follows the right hand. Arms, head, and eyes move in unison. The eyes are directed just above the outstretched right hand, gazing deep into space. The fingertips keep reaching backward and forward. Hold the posture.

3

Return to the center; briefly pause before moving in the opposite direction. The hips remain stationary; the upper torso twists. The eyes reach beyond the outstretched left hand.

Repeat at least three times before gradually increasing the pace, ultimately with swift, sweeping motions.

When bringing in rhythm, first slow down the movements before speeding up again.

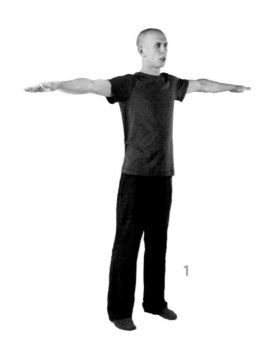

1

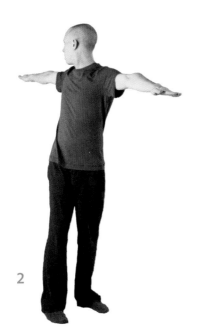

2

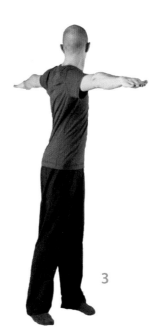

3

42

SERIES 5

The texture of human experience manifests through the senses. Whether we are working, studying, taking care of our families, or relaxing, our bodies are part of every experience, every interaction we have. Experiences of comfort, of being sick, of pleasure or pain, all are mediated by our senses. The body's five principal senses constitute our vehicle—our way of being alive. They connect us to the physical world, allowing us to find our way in space and time; they receive the world outside us on our behalf.

1

In a standing position, do a few neck rotations to loosen up the muscles of the neck. Whenever you encounter tense and painful areas, briefly hold and bring the breath there. When you are ready, turn the head to the right as far as possible. Then tilt the head slightly back, with the chin up a bit. Open the mouth and form a wide circle with your lips. The eyes are open as far as possible. The facial expression portrays something between surprise and fear.

2

Relax the eyes and mouth as you return to the center before reversing the posture. Hold this position for the same amount of time.

After completing the series, remain in stillness, without 'doing' anything.

Repeat at least three times before bringing in rhythm.

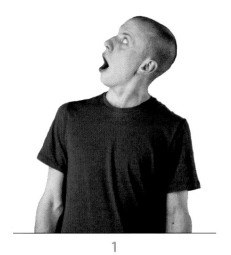

1

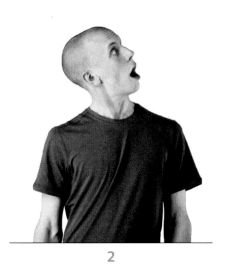

2

We can open up the depth and complexity of a single moment of feeling, gently penetrating the layers of a single sensation. When we massage the body's tissues, we can feel how our response to the touch of our hand gradually opens up: the feeling changes as tension is released. In the same way, we can massage our perceptions, our feelings, memories, and thoughts. We can explore the subtle layers of our response to a single color, how that color is woven into the fabric of our sense of self.

1

Stand with the arms at your sides, your feet firmly planted on the ground. With the whole body engaged, open the eyes a little more than you are inclined to.

2

The head turns to the right, stretching the left side of the neck. Seeing takes in all of the space it traverses through. Briefly hold the posture, allowing new sensations to arise.

3

Return to the center; the eyes follow. Minimizing the gaps in seeing-awareness, turn the head all the way to the left, stretching the right side of the neck. Briefly hold the posture.

When you are ready, switch back and forth between 2 and 3, shaking your head as if saying, 'No, no, no!'

4

Return to the center; briefly hold before tilting the head upward and slightly back. Repeat at least three times. Once the movementes are fluid, give attention to rhythm and timing.

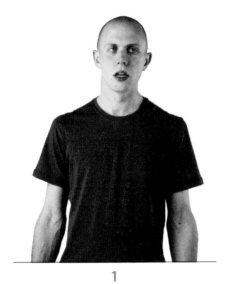

1

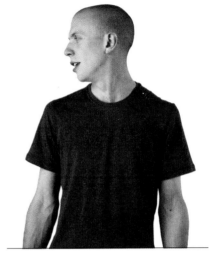

2

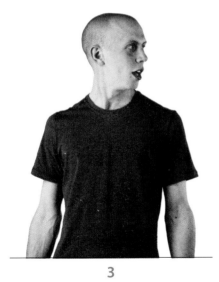

3

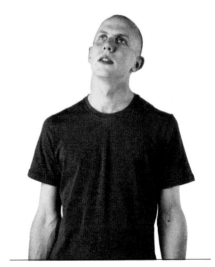

4

44

SERIES 5

Kum Nye postures penetrate the roots of experience. Gradually, we learn to distinguish where blockages are imminent and how to apply the proper antidotes. Kum Nye illuminates the various layers of experience, massaging them and bringing new relationships to light. As we work gently and precisely with the body, awareness merges with it and hidden treasures emerge. Attuning to and opening up subtle layers of presence is the essence of Kum Nye practice.

1

Bring the arms up and cross them in front of the heart chakra, the hands securely gripping the forearms. Allow the field of feelings within to merge with the posture. The eyes are wide open.

2

Lower the chin and start rotating clockwise with awareness of movement, bodily grip and direction of eyes. Moving the head and sensing each section of the neck will open the throat chakra.

3-5

As you rotate head and neck first clockwise, then counterclockwise, look ahead clearly and directly, letting the line of sight change with the movement of the head. Rotating and seeing are linked. At first, practice this movement in stages, resting after each shift; later, practice in rhythmic, continuous movements at least three times, both clockwise and counterclockwise.

⁖

44

SERIES 5

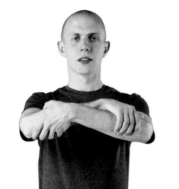

1

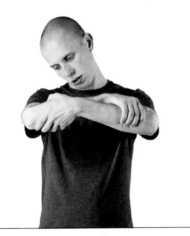

2

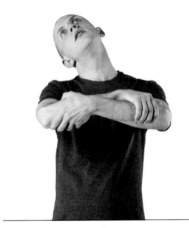

3

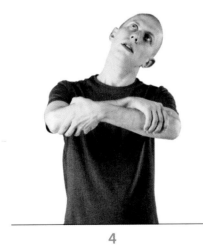

4

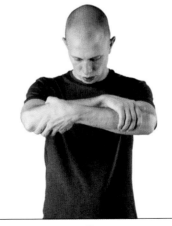

5

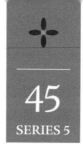

Kum Nye practice can become an opportunity to develop a deep knowledge of our individual embodiment, the specific expression of sacred energy called 'myself.'

1

Stand tall and bring body-awareness from the top of the head to the base of the feet, left and right, front and back. Make strong fists, holding them in front of the abdominal region. The hands should rest just above the navel, almost touching each other. Gaze strongly in front of you.

2

While intently and intensively holding the posture and the gaze, turn the head and move the eyes to the right. Hold the posture for a specific, predetermined length of time.

3

Turn the head back, and briefly pausing at the center before continuing in the opposite direction. Hold this posture for the same duration before returning back to center. This side-to-side movement is more than a linear progression of poses.

All movements and positions are performed rhythmically and evenly, with equal emphasis on head, eyes, and the power contained in the fists.

Repeat three times on each side before bringing in rhythm.

45
SERIES 5

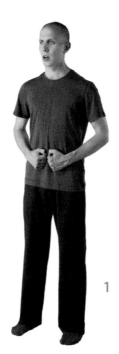

1

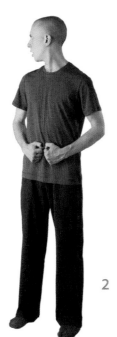

2

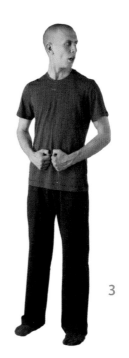

3

As we work with the positions and gestures of Kum Nye, we may find ourselves holding a pose, even when we believe we are natural. Posing is a form of acting; working with the body, we can begin to loosen up our identification with our habitual postures, our posing as ourselves. These frozen attitudes manifest our rigidity of feeling; releasing the tension that holds these poses in place also releases feeling. Kum Nye introduces us to dramatically different physical gestures. Blocked emotions melt—posing itself is liberated.

1

In a standing position, make the hands into tight fists; bend your elbows sideways and up, so the fists can move up into the armpits, with the knuckles pressing in. Look with a panoramic vision.

2

Turn the upper torso to the right. The head and the eyes follow, taking in all degrees of space. Hold the posture as you press your knuckles into the armpits. At first this area may be tender, but continued practice massages these points, transforming the experience into smooth calmness.

3

Return to center, and move on to the right. Seeing takes in all of space. Maintain pressure on the armpits and upper chest, while the entire body remains fully engaged.

Repeat three or nine times on each side, moving at the same speed, holding each position for the same amount of time. When you are ready, give particular attention to rhythm and timing.

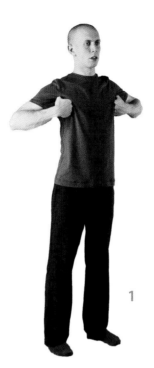

1

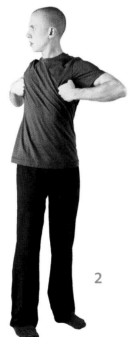

2

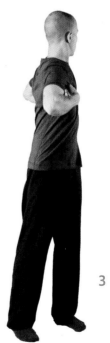

3

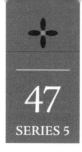

Is it possible that we could be creators of our own experience? Could we learn to manifest beauty and happiness, instead of waiting for it to be delivered to us by circumstance?

1

Before you begin, bring yourself together as a mind/body unit. Standing tall and grounded in 360-degree awareness, raise the arms in front of the body to shoulder height, palms facing each other. The eyes look straight ahead and the gaze is stable. With the arms extended, awareness of the space between the hands is activated.

2

Lift the right arm straight up, with the palm facing forward and fingertips pointing at the sky. The right hand is slightly cupped, and the eyes are directed into space on the left side of the right hand. At the same time, bring the left hand straight down to your side, keeping it slightly cupped, with the palm facing out to the left, away from the body.

3

Continuously and fluidly, without gaps in sensory awareness, allow the arms to return to shoulder height with the palms facing each other.

4

This time, the left arm moves up, the palm facing forward while the right arm and hand move downward in synchronicity with the left.

Repeat each phase of the posture with a smooth, even rhythm, three, nine or twenty-five times. Experiment with speeding up. Then bring in rhythm.

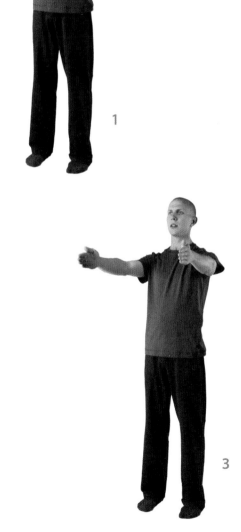

1

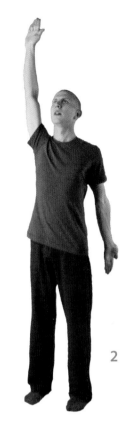

2

47

SERIES 5

3

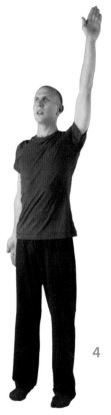

4

Body and mind coordinating, senses in harmony, free to express a myriad of characters and potentials, we begin to experience our human embodiment as a kind of choreography, a dance of space.

1

In a standing position shift your weight to the right leg and, in one fluid movement, bend your upper body to a horizontal position. Spread the arms out to the sides, palms down and cupped, and lift the left leg up behind you. All toes are flexed.

2

The left foot swings gently from right to left; the leg, the trunk, the outstretched arms and the head follow the gentle sway. Swing back and forth, three times each while the right foot and leg remain stationary.

3

Bring the body and head back up, while the left leg swings out in front, with the toes pointing up. As the leg comes up, the head and upper body tilt slightly backwards. The eyes are open wide. Head, trunk, and left leg are in one line.

Return to an upright standing position while the arms remain at shoulder height, the palms facing down. Reverse the position.

Repeat the posture three times before bringing in rhythm.

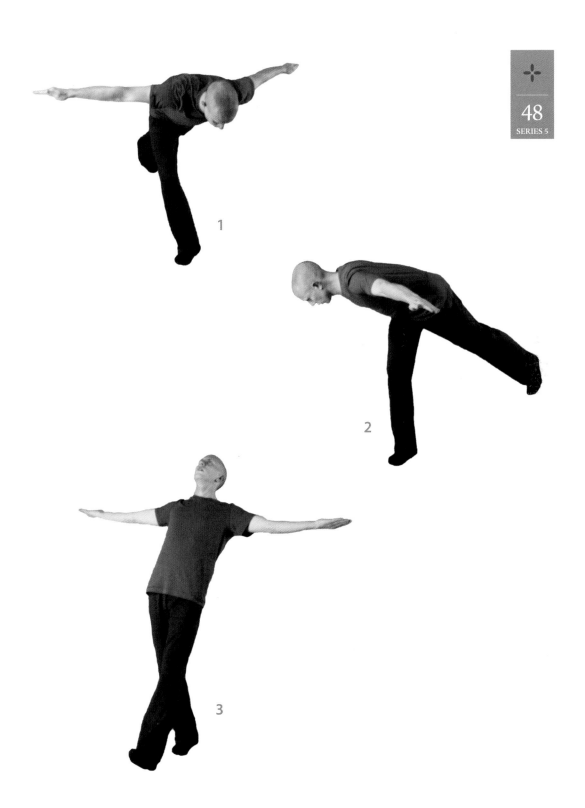

1

2

3

While we can distinguish many different levels or aspects to the human set-up, they are in reality profoundly interconnected. It is for this reason that Kum Nye practice, which can activate all the layers at once, can make deep and enduring changes in our experience.

1

In a standing position, with arms at your sides, make fists and keep them tight throughout. Cross the arms over the chest, right over left; clasp the arms closely together. The fists are placed on or near the shoulders.

2

Release the arms and open them up. The upper arms remain at shoulder height; the forearms move down horizontally, at a 90-degree angle with the upper arms. The knuckles point straight ahead.

3

Drop the elbows; the forearms come straight up, the fists stopping just above shoulder level. The elbows are not touching the body. Intensify and accumulate tension.

4

With a swift motion, thrust the arms upward with all your might, while the fists remain clenched. Stretch!

5

Release the posture. Drop the elbows; the fists stop just above the shoulder level. Push the chest forward, keeping the shoulders back. Hold the posture before repeating.

Repeat three times before bringing in rhythm.

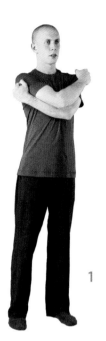

1

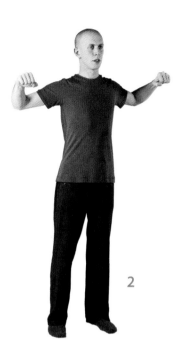

2

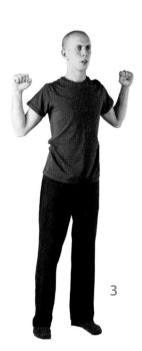

3

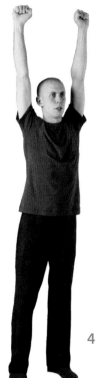

4

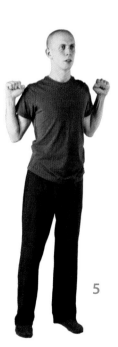

5

Kum Nye shows a way to understand what it means to be familiar with one's body. We discover that we are intimately sensing flows, fields, relations. When we make contact, we connect and that flowing quality of experience becomes part of self. Energy is making contact with energy. As energy unites with energy, another kind of consciousness can develop. Energy touching energy: this is the substance of the body's expression, the medium of knowledge manifestation.

1

In standing position, the feet at a comfortable distance apart, bend the elbows and turn the cupped hands so that the palms face upward. In front of the solar plexus, just above the navel, make an offering gesture with the cupped hands; the fingers are touching and point up, with the thumbs separate.

2

Raise both hands, fingertips touching; as they move up, turn them in front of the heart. Briefly pause with the cupped hands at upper chest level. The thumbs and palms are pointing down, the elbows are spread out to the sides.

3

Continue the hands' journey upward until they are over the head; turn the palms out and upward, with the thumbs sticking out.

4

With a grand opening gesture, the arms move to the sides with the palms down. Rather than focusing on the movement, focus on the rapport of the cupped hands and the thumbs with space.

5

The arms reach shoulder height. This is an important moment; briefly pause before you shift down, bringing new experience into standing tall.

Repeat three times before bringing in rhythm.

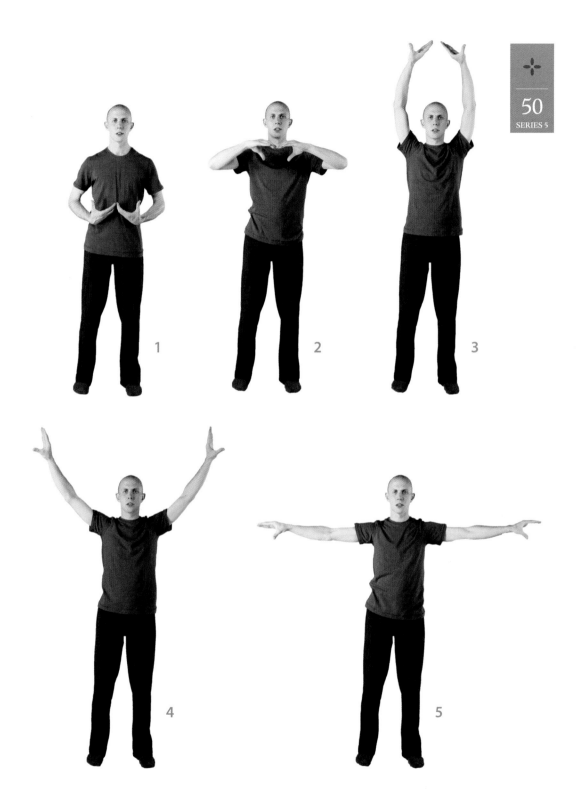

1

2

3

4

5

Works of art encourage us to look deeply at the physical world, and see it as a manifestation of sacred energies. Without this precious embodiment, without manifestation, no work of art can exist. Art depends on the body, but it also reveals the body's hidden beauty.

1

Stand tall, with full awareness from head to toe. Gathering all the energies of body and mind, cross your outstretched arms, hands and fingers in front of the body, and lower the chin to the chest. The eyes are cast down, looking within. You are embodying a unique facet of total aliveness. Hold the posture for thirty or sixty seconds, ready to 'explode' at any time into posture 2.

2

Vigorously express the opposite of the previous posture. As the heart soars, reaching higher and higher, open the arms wide at your sides, palms out, feeling energy flowing through the fingertips. Without placing strain on the neck, tilt the head back and direct the gaze deeply and widely into space. Hold the posture for the same amount of time as posture 1. Shift back and forth between the two postures, over and over again.

51
SERIES 5

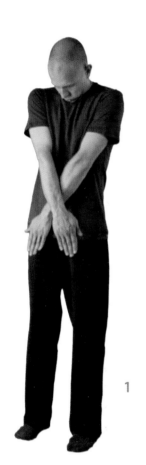

1

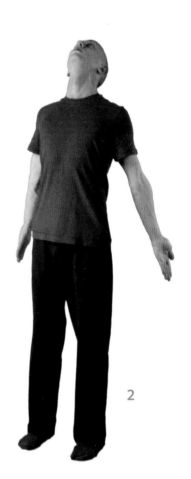

2

Concentrating lightly, we exhale, allowing each movement of our bodies to encourage and extend the flow of the breath. Each shift of position can release tension, melting the blockages we have been keeping in our feet, our joints, our backs, our bellies, necks and shoulders. Moving, breathing freely, we can untangle the knots in the stomach, soften the obstruction in the throat, and uncover the tension hidden in our faces and behind our eyes. In time, these movements can release not only physical tension, but the subtler tension of sensing, thinking, and feeling. We let go, exhale, rejoice, release. Releasing becomes ease.

1

In a standing position, place your feet hip-width apart. Put the hands on the knees with the thumbs on the inside and the fingers pointing outward. While the arms remain straight, the shoulders come up and backward. Relax the neck as the shoulders are compacting. Bend the knees and lower the buttocks. Drop the head. Hold the posture; emphasize the exhalation.

2

Straighten the legs; release the shoulders as the back and head align into a horizontal position. Hold the posture; emphasize the exhalation.

3

Release the hands. As the arms come forward and up, they lead the way for the torso and head to straighten.

4

The arms continue to rise all the way up, the cupped palms of the hands facing forward. The eyes keep looking straight ahead. Hold the posture. When you are ready, release the arms, letting them come forward and down.

Repeat three times before bringing in rhythm.

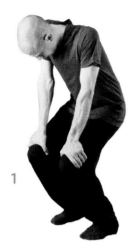

1

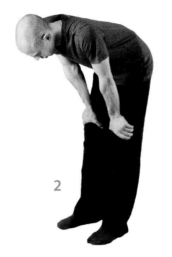

2

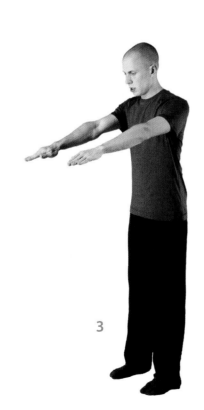

3

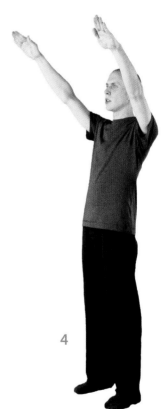

4

53

SERIES 6

With soft eyes, we touch the depths of seeing. We can make direct contact with light, something we don't always notice, because we are too busy seeing the things around us with the aid of light. Hearing and smelling, touching and tasting may be the same. It may take time and patience to excavate them, but we can develop more and more knowledge of our senses, our experience, through gentleness. And, gentleness can take us to depths of feeling that forcing cannot reach.

1

Stand tall and clasp the hands at the base of the skull. Expose the armpits; the elbows are stretched back and pointing up.

2

The upper body bends at the waist horizontally, stretching from the back of the neck to the tailbone. The top of the head is pointing forward. The elbows are pointing sideways and slightly upward.

3

In one movement bring the torso back up and raise the chest, tilting the head back. Make this upright position expressive.

Repeat three times before bringing in the rhythm.

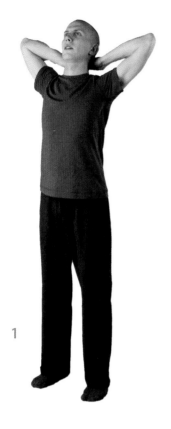

1

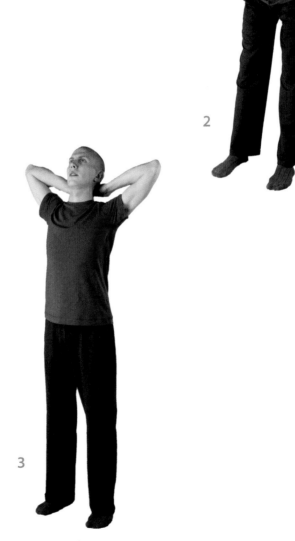

2

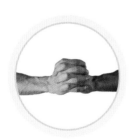

Interlaced

3

As we engage the flow of feeling, each technique, gesture, and posture becomes a form of creative expression. The movements of our bodies begin to communicate deep experiences of wholeness; our gestures manifest the alignment of body and mind.

1

In standing position, with the feet at a comfortable distance apart, interlock the fingers and place them at the base of the skull. The elbows are spread, the armpits open.

2

Bend the upper body forward into a horizontal position, with the face down. Accumulate your energy in stretching your torso and neck, not holding back, and not straining. Lightly push your hands against the base of the skull so the energy contained here can be integrated into the posture.

3

Move back into the upward position and raise your arms up, all the way over your head, stretching the interlocked hands. Release the posture by lowering the arms sideways.

Repeat all steps in a continuous motion, taking equal time for all positions and movements.

Repeat at least three times before bringing in rhythm.

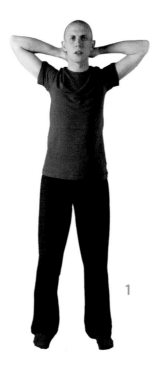

1

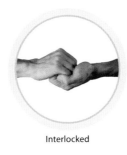

Interlocked

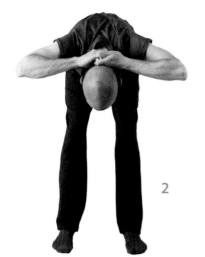

2

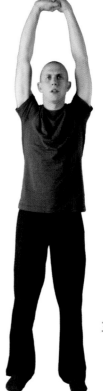

3

Kum Nye enables you to perform in the present moment without being in the mode of correcting yourself or refining yourself. There is no judgment or projection of experience. Such activities imply a separation between the corrector and what is being corrected. If the act of Kum Nye is really taking place, there is only doing; in that moment of pure activity there is no room for correction. If you do make a change, the moment of action is innocent of all judgment, comparison and correction.

1

In standing position, pull in the navel and keep it held in throughout. Tighten the fists and hold them close to the abdominal region, pulling back the shoulders and elbows. Accumulate energy in the upper body and gradually let it disperse throughout the entire body. The eyes are steady.

2

Lift the right shoulder as high as possible, moving it slightly forward; lower the left shoulder while moving it slightly backward. The torso twists to the left, but the head remains facing forward.

3

Release the posture and return to the center. Briefly pause before reversing the posture to the right. The clenched fists are in contact with the body and the energy within.

Make the movements dramatic; exaggerate the shoulder movements and the torso twists.

Repeat at least three times before bringing in rhythm.

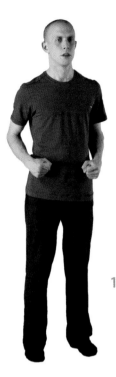

1

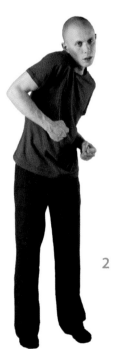

2

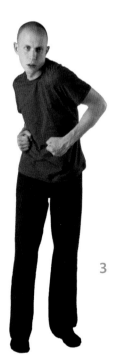

3

Relaxation, release, opens our range of motion. It becomes possible to dance. Dancing is an expression of the body's joy, a gesture that transforms ordinary movement into art. Dance salvages our suffering, represents the characters of human experience, revealing it all as beautiful and meaningful.

1

In standing position, place the feet hip-width apart. The arms are alongside the body, and the hands remain cupped throughout. The fingers are held together, lightly touching the surface of the body. Notice how the sensations arising from this contact are changing in each moment.

2

The right arm moves up straight ahead, with the hand facing in. When the hand approaches shoulder height, the eyes make a connection with it, looking past the palm into the distance. The fingertips are piercing space.

3

The eyes remain aligned with the right palm and beyond, as the arm continues its journey all the way up. The head tilts backward as the eyes follow the hand.

4

The right arm continues to travel backward and down, and the shoulder and head turn accordingly. Throughout the gesture, remain in contact with the unmoving left palm. As the cycle is being completed, the head and shoulder return to the center. Without interruption, reverse and begin lifting the left arm.

Repeat the complete cycle at least three times before bringing in rhythm.

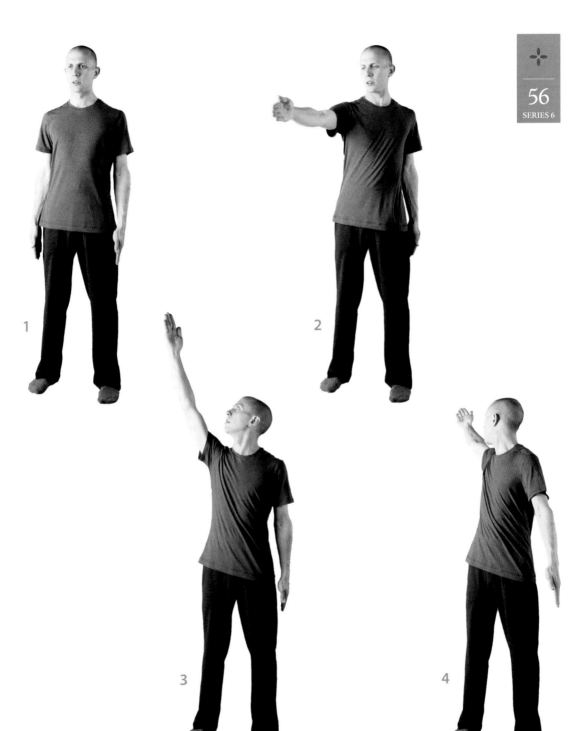

1

2

3

4

57

SERIES 6

Layer by layer, our sense perceptions, thoughts and feelings can be transformed. Each sensation has subtle gradations and shifts within it. Yet the deeper we go, the more we relax into the sensation, the more open and spacious the sensation itself becomes. We can explore these layers by working with a single exercise over time.

1

Stand tall, with the feet a comfortable distance apart, about the width of your hips. Raise the arms straight in front to shoulder height, with the palms facing each other. Look in a panoramic way.

2

As the right arm moves up, the head turns to the right and the eyes look beyond the arm, deep into space. The left arm moves downward and reaches back as far as possible. Both hands face inward.

3

When the right arm moves down, the left comes up, and both arms meet in front of the heart, before continuing in the opposite directions.

4

The left arm goes up all the way, while the right arm moves down, reaching backward as far as possible.

Once you are familiar with these movements, increase the speed from slow to medium, and then as fast as you can, almost chaotically. The eyes do not go blank as they sweep from side to side; maintain rapport with seeing in space.

Continue, bringing in rhythm, even when increasing speed to a maximum.

⋱⋰

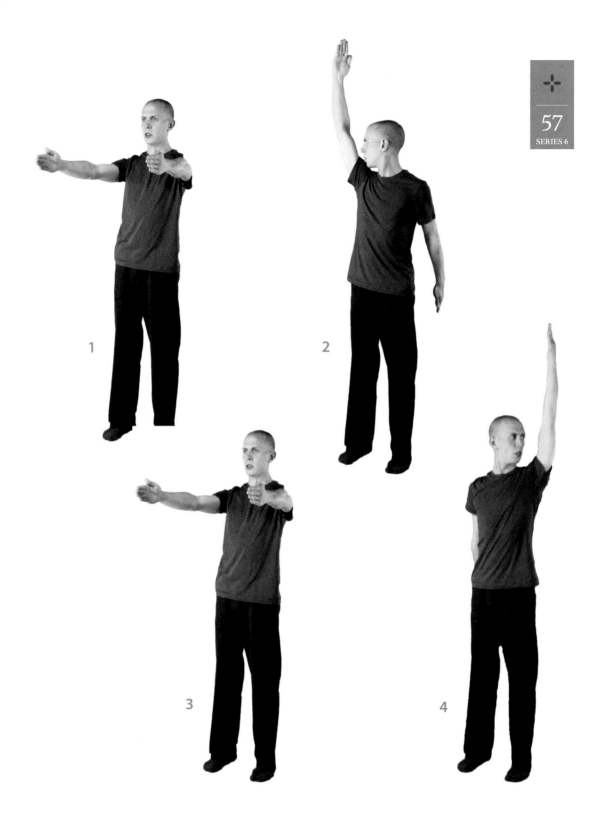

1

2

3

4

Kum Nye training can bring to light your expression of energy, your specific embodiment, and your moment in time, giving you knowledge that ultimately there is a reason for your being here, for your undertaking this journey. You have a purpose. And your purpose may be up to you!

1

Stand straight, with the arms alongside the body. Take time to gather the energy to make firm fists. The gaze is open, yet determined; look ahead. Lift the right knee at a 90-degree angle to the ground and flex the foot; briefly hold.

2

While the entire body is grounded in the left leg, kick the right foot forward, straightening the leg and keeping the toes flexed. Hold the posture for the same amount of time as 1. Express your energy! Bring the right foot down, holding the fists tight.

3

Reverse the posture, and shift the weight to the right leg, maximally tightening the fists. Now lift the left leg, foot flexed, and hold. There is a correlation between the determined look in the eyes, the firm fists, the tension in the raised foot, and this moment in time. Ready to explode in the next pose?

4

Kick the left leg forward with total purpose; the eyes, fists and foot are all aligned in this abrupt movement. Hold the posture. Return to the stationary position and release the hands.

Repeat three times before bringing in rhythm.

At the end of each cycle, open the hands and stand tall.

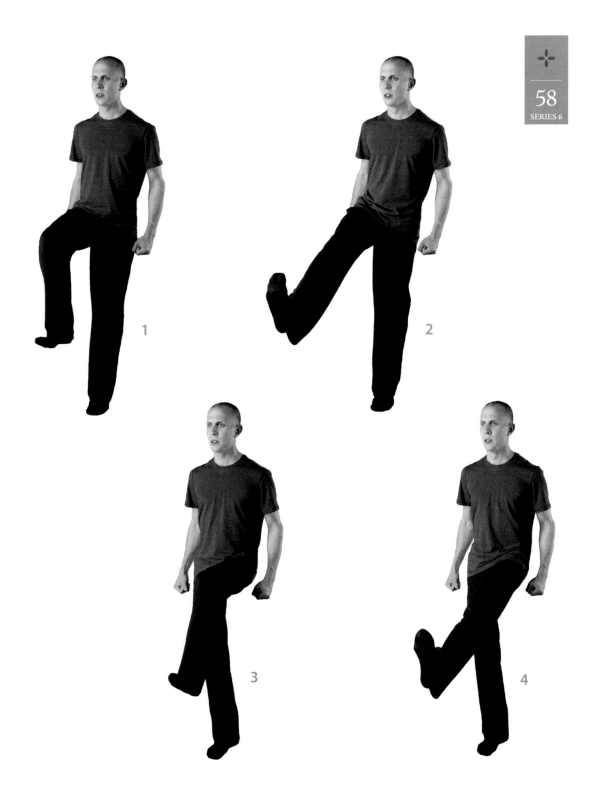

1

2

3

4

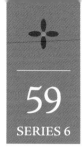

As you work more closely with the positions and gestures of Kum Nye, you may find yourself holding a pose even if you think you are being natural. Just as the actor is different from the role, you too can begin to loosen up your identification with your habitual postures, your posing as your self.

1

Stand tall, the feet close together. The arms and legs are engaged; the body is poised, ready to move.

2

Raise the left arm forward to shoulder height, with the hand cupped, the palm facing inward. At the same time, the left leg vigorously steps to the right, with flexed toes, crossing over the right leg as far as possible. The eyes follow and the torso turns to the right, with the outstretched arm sweeping through space. You may be on the verge of losing balance. During this stride through space, the right arm comes up and the cupped hand, facing inward, crosses the solar plexus, reaching to the left at a 90-degree angle with the outstretched arm. Return to the center and release the posture.

3

Reverse the posture. The right arm comes up in front, with the palm cupped. The left arm is still at the side. The right leg moves to the left as far as it can, crossing over the left leg, with the toes flexed; at the same time the left arm comes up and passes over the solar plexus, reaching with cupped hand and piercing fingers as the torso turns to the left. In this position, to stagger or sway is better than to hold back.

Repeat at least three times before bringing in rhythm.

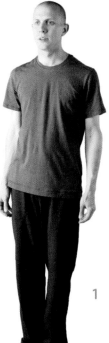

1

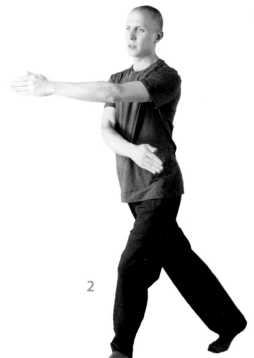

2

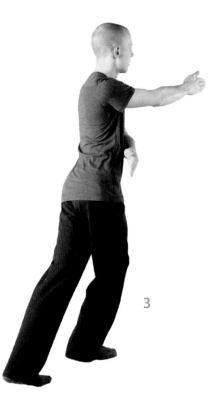

3

When we practice Kum Nye in this way, it becomes more than a set of exercises or ideas. It becomes a mode of inquiry, a space in which we are free to notice the mounting of the production, discovering the subtle operations of our senses, the profound effects of language and culture upon the ways of being we normally take for granted.

1

In standing position, emphasize exhaling a few times. Then the left arm comes up forward and the right arm moves up backward; they are aligned at approximately a 30-degree angle. The palms are cupped. The body and the head remain facing forward throughout. Briefly hold the posture. The breath is as light as possible and might even seem absent at times.

2

The arms come down, passing the hips at the same time before moving into the opposite direction. Once you are familiar with the movement, the speed may increase; the entire body is engaged as the arms are swishing through space.

Slow down and come to a halt with one arm straight ahead, and the other arm backward, before lowering both arms.

Then start again for nine or twenty-five cycles, bringing in rhythm.

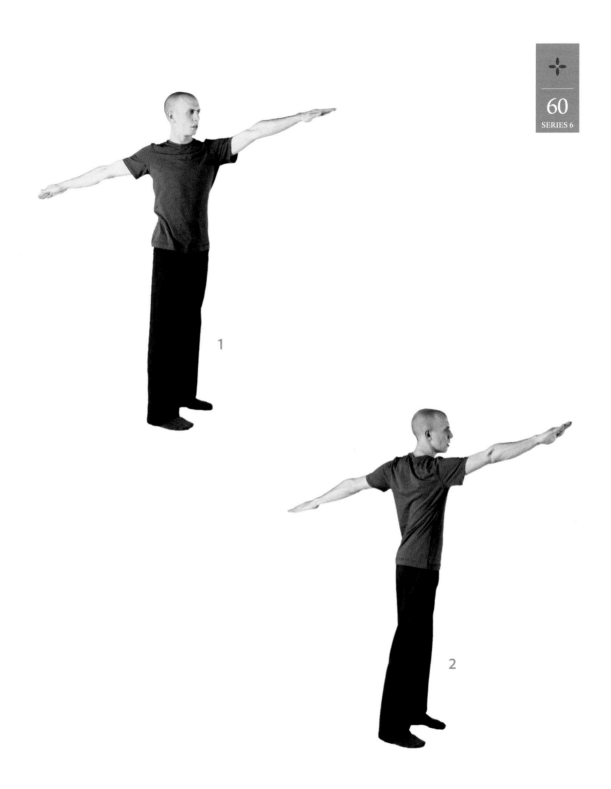

When we have gained unshakeable confidence in wholeness, we cannot help but share our experience with others, for it shines in us, in our bodies, our minds, and our actions.

1

While standing comfortably, take time to cultivate awareness in the entire body. Feel how the feet are rooted in the earth, the arms are hanging at your sides.

2

Raise the arms in front of the body and then over the head, until the fingers are pointing backward, with the palms flat. Sense the stretch along the insides of the arms and through the underarms.

3-4

Twist the upper body to the left and bend down to a horizontal position, stretching all the way from the tailbone to the fingertips. Then the upper body passes in a sweeping motion through the center to the other side. The fingertips, hands and arms keep reaching as the movement continues to the right, until the torso cannot stretch any further.

5

Still in the horizontal plane, move back to the center and lower the arms, flexing the wrists. Slightly bend the knees and let the palms almost touch the ground, but not quite. The head stays parallel to the ground, in a smooth line with the neck and spine. Straighten the legs, stretching the hips back and upward. Lift the hands to knee level, palms still facing down. Pause briefly. Continue to rise until you have returned to the upright position.

Repeat the sequence three or nine times in rhythm, mindful of how the wide-open eyes sweep through every part of space.

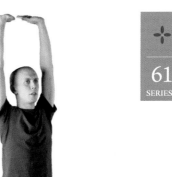

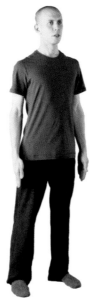

1

2

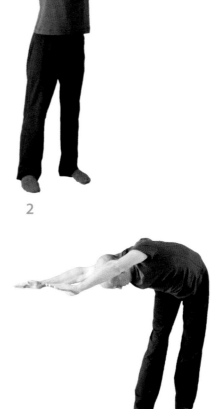

3

4

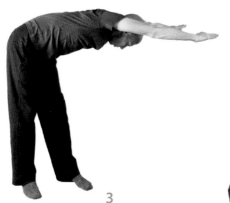

5

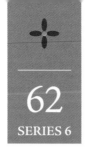

62

SERIES 6

Great practitioners foster a positive relationship between the outside world and their senses. Open and pure, embracing their surroundings without judgment, they find deep contentment and beauty even in difficult circumstances. We too can engage experience in transformative ways; our practice can lead to a heightened appreciation of the wondrous beauty of being. Kum Nye practice is an approach that allows us to discover that significance fills every experience; each can become a work of art. As we practice Kum Nye, we can develop creativity as a way of being.

1

Stand tall and raise the arms in front of you, at shoulder height, with the palms facing each other. Slowly begin stretching the left arm out and slightly upward, while turning the left hand, which is cupped, until the palm faces forward. Meanwhile, the right arm bends and the hand moves back until it stops at the shoulder. The right palm is facing outward. The body is turned in such a way that the arms form one line. The eyes look into space, their gaze brushing the thumb of the outstretched hand. The view is both broad and deep.

2

Switch sides. Switching has the quality of a ritual; the arms are delicately tuned in a way that would captivate an outside observer.

Alternate the postures three times on each side. Then add rhythm.

⋱⋰

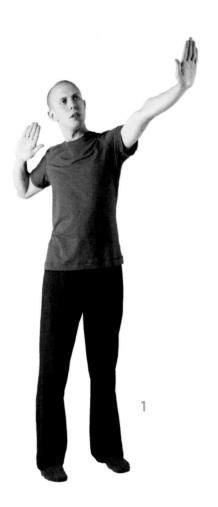

1

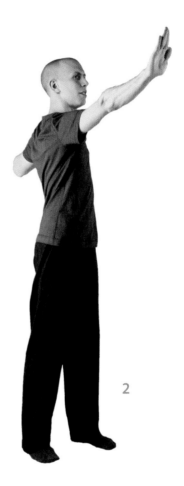

2

The work of yoga might be seen as joining up two distinct entities, 'body' and 'mind.' Yet Kum Nye practice is a process by which intimate relations are revealed. The closer we look, the harder it is to find a firm separation of body and mind. Because of our limited concepts and experience of body and mind, we might miss the energy at play within us. Kum Nye may seem like practices performed by and for the body, but each posture, each movement reflects this play of subtle energy. The release of tension frees up this energy and lets it move naturally: body and mind together dance and play.

1

Sit in the seven gestures or in the lotus position. Put your fists at the crease between the torso and the thighs, digging the knuckles in. Breathe deeply, directing the air down through the central column of the body to a point just above the base of the trunk, below the navel. Hold the breath and keep it there as long as possible. Look with a panoramic gaze and simultaneously straight ahead, with strong intention.

2

While you are still holding the breath, straighten the arms, intensifying the posture. Imagine you are sitting on top of the breath. Hold the breath a little longer than you may be inclined to. Then, let it go gradually, exhaling and releasing the shoulders and arms into the first pose. The breath flows freely. The energy moves naturally.

When you are ready, repeat the posture and breathing pattern at least twice.

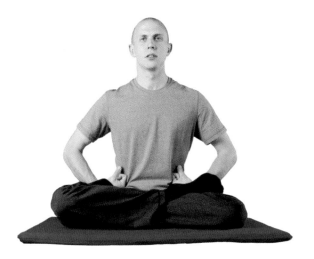

1

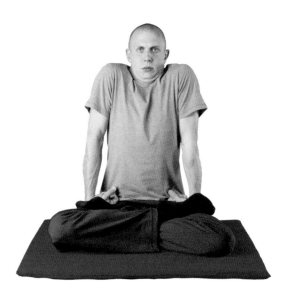

2

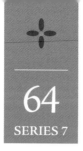

64

SERIES 7

Think of Kum Nye practice as a form of knowledge-gathering, in a spirit of open inquiry. You are acquiring knowledge you did not have before. The body is not the object of study; instead, it is an active partner with which to experience the wonder of really getting to know your self from the inside out. This exploration offers the gift of a lived awareness, and knowing becomes a form of intimacy with all you experience.

1

Getting ready: gather the field of energy within the body. Place the hands just above the knees, thumbs inward. Bend the knees, push down to the spot that stirs the most energy and hold.

2

Straighten the body and raise the arms to shoulder height, with the cupped hands facing down, while spreading the legs wide.

3

The left arm moves forward and the right arm backward, forming a straight line. The upper body twists to the right. The head follows the right hand and the eyes sweep through space, all the way back.

4

Reverse the pose, moving the right arm forward and the left backward. The head follows the left hand.

5

Pause in the center with the arms at shoulder height. Raise the arms overhead; the hands are cupped, palms facing forward.

After three or nine repetitions, 3 and 4 are repeated nine or twenty-five times at a higher speed.

∴

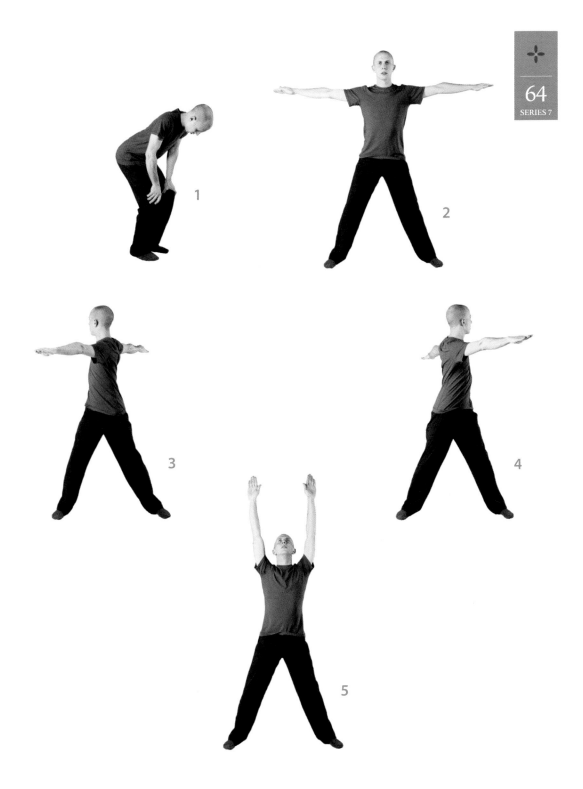

1

2

3

4

5

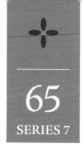

65

SERIES 7

Our experiences are not unlike the various manifestations of water. Snow, ice, rain, waves, and streams are all expressions of water. Similarly, thoughts, sensations, and emotional states can all be understood as expressions of a basic, fundamental openness. Through Kum Nye we can sense the ripples of experiences forming, spreading, and dispersing again, smoothing away into calmness. Working with the Kum Nye postures, we can penetrate the nature of experience and enter an open field of awareness.

1

Raise the arms in front of the torso, the palms facing upward as if holding space.

2

Together the arms move in the same plane to the right, stimulating feelings and holding the posture with fervor.

3

Move back, briefly pause at the center and continue to the left, stirring up more feeling. Continue back and forth, pausing each time in the middle, at the right and at the left for equal amounts of time.

With each movement, let mind settle more deeply. As you bring in rhythm, the separation between experiencer and experience dissolves.

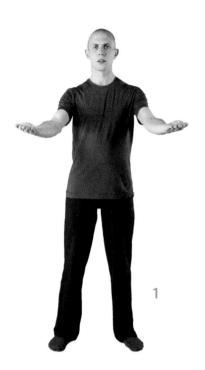

1

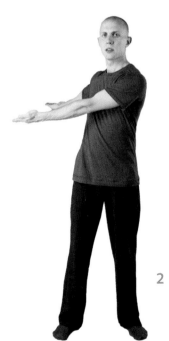

2

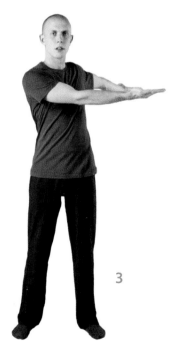

3

Kum Nye can have a powerful impact on our being human. We can allow freedom of movement to ourselves, to our experience of being 'I.' Obstacles and blockages that seem carved in stone, just the way things have to be, begin to disclose their developmental paths, in the process losing their hardness. The more closely we look at these phenomena, the more apparent it becomes that all these seemingly permanent structures—even the 'I' itself—are expressions of energy.

1

Stretch out the right arm, slightly cupping the hand and pointing the fingers down at a 45-degree angle with the ground. Cross the left arm over the heart with the palm facing up. The head follows the movement of the outstretched arm; the eyes continue in the direction where the fingertips are pointing.

2

Lift up the arms, hands and eyes and continue the circular movement. The eyes look alongside the outstretched arm, past the fingertips, deep into space.

3

Both arms reach upward, above the head, with fingertips pointing straight up. The eyes gaze into the depth of the sky.

4

Continue the circular movement of the hands toward the left. The left arm points up to the left, while the right hand forms the offering support.

5

Arms, hands, and eyes go down, and move through the center to 1.

As you bring in rhythm, experiment with slowing down and speeding up.

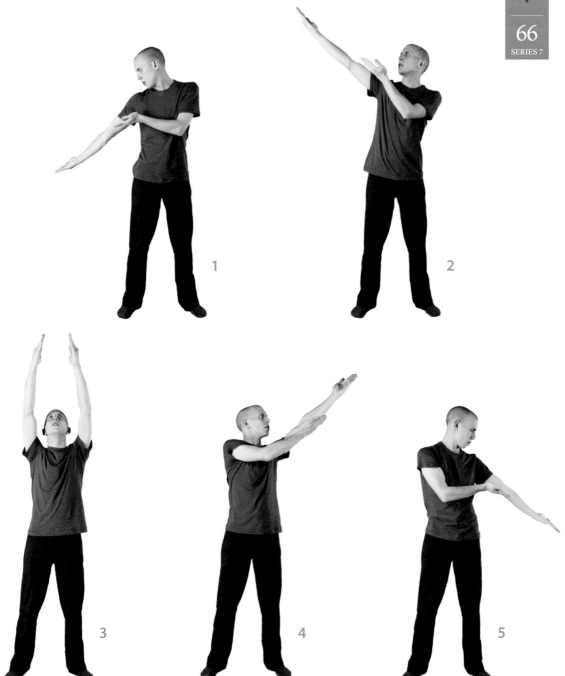

1

2

3

4

5

The interplay between mind and body is far from simple; the human set-up has many layers that work together to produce even our most basic and mundane experiences. When our minds and bodies coordinate, we are comfortable, healthy, and happy.

1

Raise the arms at the sides to shoulder height, with the palms slightly cupped, facing down. Shift your weight to the left leg and raise the right foot, lifting the toes upward. Make sure you are grounded on the stationary leg all the way up along that side of the body. At first you may be wobbly. After a while, there is no difference whether the leg is on or off the ground. Let the right knee bend slightly outward. Hold the posture for a predetermined time—for example, for four counts.

2

Keeping the arms at shoulder height, lower the right leg. Take the same amount of time for this movement as in 1. Now, shift your weight to the right side in preparation for lifting the left leg. When the left leg comes up, let it cross slightly over the stationary leg before turning it up and out toward the left; there is a gentle swing to this movement.

Hold the posture for the same amount of time before lowering it, at the same pace. Place both feet on the ground for the same four counts; this is not a rest, but an integral part of the movement.

Repeat nine or twenty-five times, in one expressive rhythm.

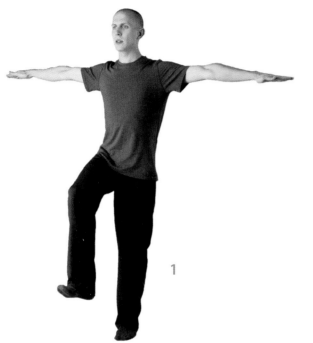

1

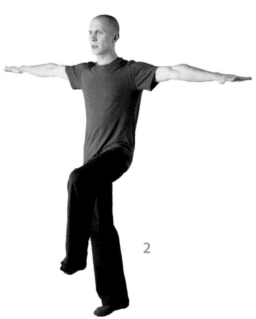

2

Kum Nye has the power to affect our energy levels and our physical and mental flexibility. The postures open startling alternatives to our ordinary approaches to life, which are hardened into place by years of repetition. They generate an effect that is felt at the energy and feeling level. By intensifying bodily experience through movement and posture, Kum Nye addresses impacted parts of the self directly and decisively.

1

Place the feet at a comfortable distance apart. Lift the arms forward and up. Keeping the elbows straight, interlace the fingers and turn the hands so that the palms face upward. Look with panoramic vision.

2

Shift your weight to the left leg and bring the right knee up; the foot is flexed and the toes point upward.

3

Stretch the upper body and the arms to the left, extending as far as you can without straining the left side of the rib cage, as the arms and the hands keep reaching.

Return to the center, with both feet on the floor. The arms are released forward and down. Reverse the posture, shifting to the right leg.

Repeat three times on each side. Once the movements and transitions are fluid, bring in rhythm.

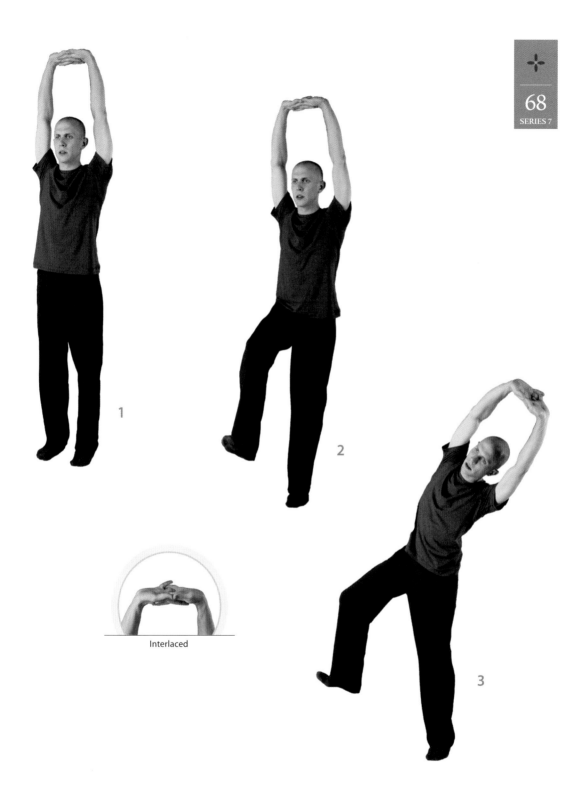

1

Interlaced

2

3

Kum Nye helps to contact various dimensions of experience; your sense of identity begins to shift at its core. The practices can loosen the bonds of habit and assumption, opening up restrictive orientations of perceptions, body, and mind. None of the postures has an emotional tone. As the mind grows steadier, thinking no longer poses an obstacle to being. The nucleus of the self opens up; as energy is released, unexpected treasures emerge.

1

Lift the arms sideways to shoulder height, in a straight line, with the palms facing down.

2

Keeping the arms at shoulder height, move them to the front of the body and turn the palms upward.

3

Lift the arms straight over the head, wrists bent, palms facing upward, assembling all energies in the upward movement.

4

Bring body, mind, senses, and space awareness into this pose. Bring the arms forward, palms facing down and fingertips pointing straight ahead. The hands are slightly cupped. Bend at the knees to stir up maximum lower body energy.

5

Turn the cupped palms up and out. Vigorously swing the right arm back while emphatically stretching the left arm forward. The head follows the hand that is pointing backward. Switch the positions of the arms, each time holding the posture for a moment. Fiercely switch back and forth ten or twenty-five times. At the end, let the arms return to the sides and stand tall before moving on or sitting down.

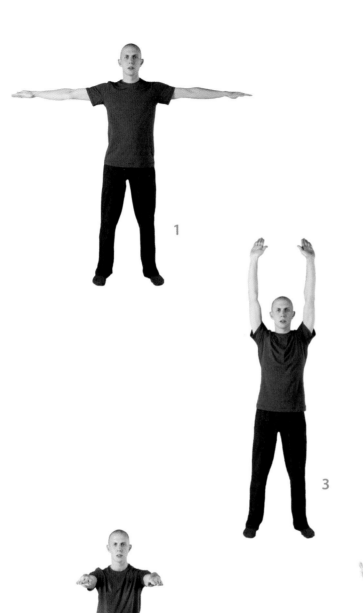

1

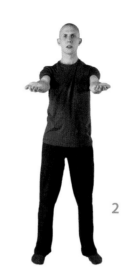

2

3

4

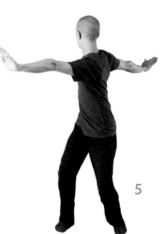

5

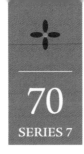

70

SERIES 7

Even though they dwelled in austere, even harsh places, the great yogis of history were highly developed internally; they were constantly enjoying every drop of their living experience. They rejoiced in the sounds they heard, the flavors they tasted, the odors they smelled, the textures they touched, and the light they perceived. They were artists without a canvas; their way of being in the world was their masterpiece, and even their most ordinary gestures and expressions could conduct creativity. As we practice Kum Nye dancing, we can do this in our own ways.

1

Begin by grounding yourself. Raise your arms in front of you to shoulder height, with the palms facing down. As your weight shifts to the left, simultaneously raise the heel of the right foot and the right arm.

2

Keeping your weight settled on the left foot, flex the right foot, and lift the right knee and right arm in the same motion. The toes point up, the knee goes up, as the arm rises. Joyfully move the arm and leg up and down in a smooth rhythm. Touch the ground with the toes before lifting the leg again, stirring up space on the right side.

3

Bring both arms back to the front, parallel to each other. Shift your weight to the right, and repeat the same movement with the left leg and arm. Each round has the same duration.

Repeat the gesture on each side three or nine times, experimenting with speeding up the movement slightly. Once the movements are fluid, bring in rhythm.

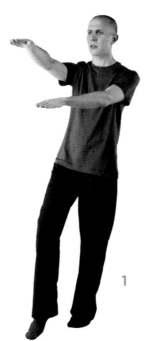

1

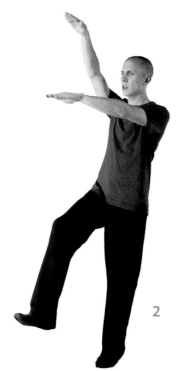

2

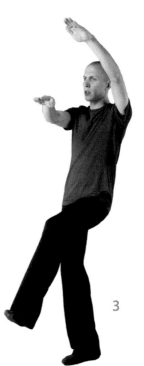

3

According to the Kum Nye tradition, a healthy mind inhabits the present moment. Undisturbed by memories of the past, free of fears in the present, and unconcerned with projections of the future, a healthy mind engages experience freshly and directly. The present moment is the moment of embodiment—the right now of experience.

1

Place the feet a comfortable distance apart, the weight equally distributed on the balls of both feet. Assembling all energy and focus, bring the arms straight in front, hands slightly cupped, and palms facing down.

In one fluent motion, raise the left leg; bend the knee, briefly crossing it over the standing leg before swinging it all the way to the left. The foot lands as far away as possible, in a 90-degree angle, while the torso turns to the left as well. Now shift your weight even further forward onto the left knee, and while the torso remains erect, straighten the right leg behind you, with the foot still in the starting position.

Simultaneously, the left arm is raised at a 45-degree angle. The palm is directed forward and the fingers are pointing to the ceiling; meanwhile, the right arm swings backward, the palm facing down. Both arms are aligned. The gaze looks up and ahead, just brushing the thumb of the outstretched left hand.

2

Reverse, and repeat three or nine times; then add rhythm.

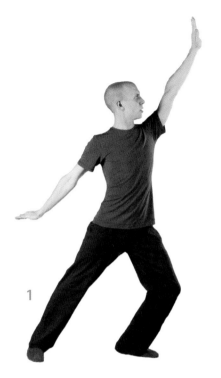

1

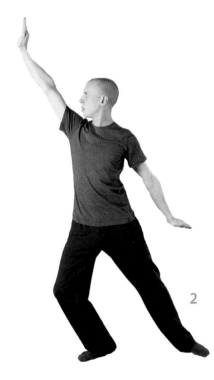

2

How can we access the nourishment available in the present moment? We sense that relaxation is the key. Relaxation is a state of being we could call dynamic rest. Calm and flowing, peaceful yet alert, true relaxation expresses itself both in movement and in stillness.

1

Stand tall and still, dynamically at rest. Prepare to move clockwise. Shift your weight to the left leg; in unison the right arm and right leg come up high while the left arm moves back, stretched behind the body. The palms of the hands are cupped; the right palm faces forward, while the left palm is turned slightly upward. The lifted foot is flexed, the toes pointing upward. Look with a panoramic gaze.

2

The transitions matter; bring in a quality of grace and resolve. In one continuous motion, switch the positions of arms, legs and feet, while moving in a circle clockwise, taking small steps.

3

As you continue to turn to the right, allow yourself to be engaged within; not bracing yourself, but free to move. The gaze traverses space mindfully.

Repeat at least three times before experimenting with bringing in rhythm and speeding up. Express the union of mind and body in a continuous motion.

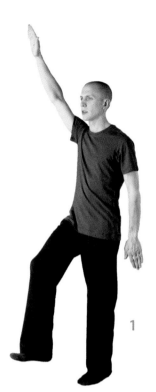

1

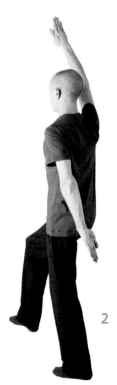

2

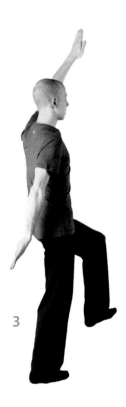

3

When the energy of human embodiment is fully expressed, it becomes art. It reveals our inner qualities, our distinctive flavors, our souls. We become one with joy; the expression of joy is our dancing.

1

Raise the arms sideways to shoulder height. The right arm is outstretched and points slightly upwards, while the left arm bends at the elbow, which is slightly pointing down. Bring the left wrist close to the left shoulder and push the elbow backward. The palm of the left hand faces forward, the palm of the right hand faces to the right. The middle and ring fingers of both hands are touching the thumb, and the index and little finger point straight up.

Place the feet at a 90-degree angle to each other, wide apart. The right foot is in line with the right arm and the left foot points in the same direction as the left hand. The eyes and the head follow the outstretched arm.

Now shift your weight onto the left leg, bending the left knee while firmly straightening the right leg. Shift your balance all the way back.

2

Bend the right knee and shift your weight to the right leg. Bend both knees further until you contact and explosive point.

3

With the arms and hands in the same skillful position, jump up, both feet off the ground. Pull up the knees as high as possible while the toes point down, in a single explosion of energy. Land on the balls of your feet; move three hops forward and two hops back. Repeat this series of hops three times.

Reverse the posture. Add rhythm.

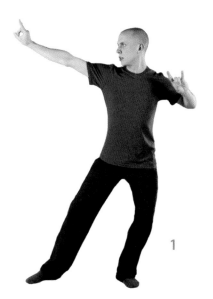

1

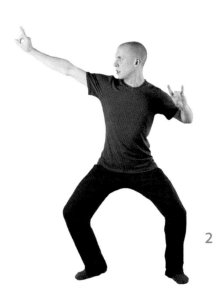

2

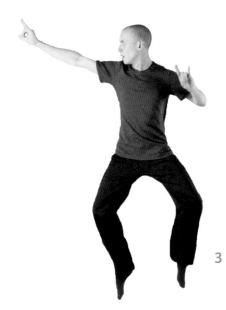

3

What is Kum Nye's ultimate purpose? Perhaps to help human beings make direct contact with their part in the field of being, their purpose. This purpose is as unique and individual as a fingerprint; like the depth of bodily knowledge, it can not easily be codified, but can be freely expressed, in movement and stillness, in gesture and action.

1

Stretch the left arm forward and up, and the right arm backward so that they form a straight line at a 45-degree angle. Throughout this posture the hands are cupped. The left palm faces forward, and the right is directed toward the ground. The left leg and arm are lifted at the same time; the toes are flexed.

2

As you raise your left knee, compact your trunk and shift your weight to the toes of the rigth leg. Feel how your body is getting ready to jump. Now the right leg takes off and jumps in the air, pulling up the right knee as high as possible.

Reverse by shifting your weight to the left leg. The right arm goes up, the left arm reaches backward, in a straight line at a 45-degree angle.

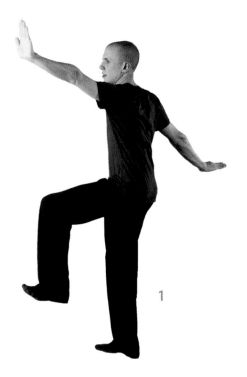

1

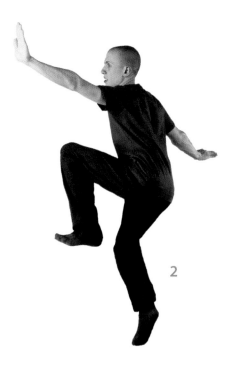

2

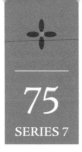

As we continue, eventually we can treat all practice as a continuous release of tension, conducting us to greater and greater ease. Ultimately, we are not just practicing one exercise, one pose at a time. Swimming has individual strokes, distinctive motions—but swimming itself is a smooth, continuous movement through the water. Our gestures gradually acquire this connected quality as we practice: body movements become a kind of floating in ease.

1

In a standing position, place the feet at a comfortable distance apart. Make fists and raise the arms, crossing them in front of the chest with the knuckles pointing behind you. The elbows are pointing straight ahead. Tighten the posture, especially the arms and fists, but also the belly area. Accumulate and compact the energy, as if you were ready to burst.

2

Abruptly open the arms and let them fall to the sides at 45-degree angles, the fists opening into cupped hands. The posture is released all at once, as if your heart opens wide.

Alternate between the two positions, briefly holding each. Throughout, the eyes look straight ahead with a kind gaze.

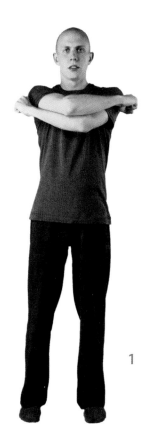

1

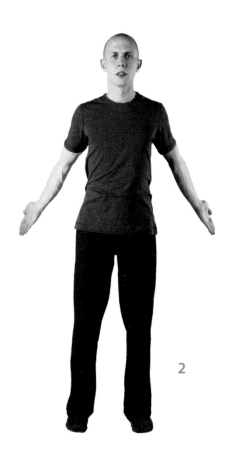

2

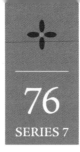

When we truly recognize that our experience is fundamentally open and flexible, we are free to respond creatively. As we become masters of our own experience, we can replant the gardens of our minds. We can rekindle the joy of past experience, allowing its energy to mingle with and transform the quality of the present experience.

With the heels touching, come up onto the balls of the feet. Raise the arms sideways to shoulder height, with the fingertips pointing down and the palms cupped. Bending the knees slightly, move up and down a few times, until you touch a point that holds the most impact or power. Allow the movement to express openness and flexibility. Look with a panoramic vision, wide and sharp at the same time.

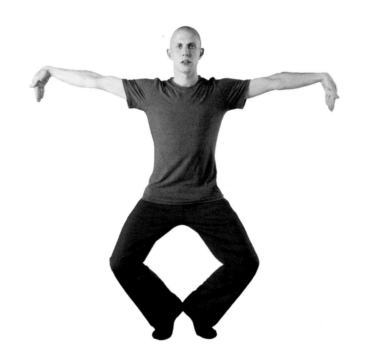

DANCING A MYSTERY

The Kum Nye dance expresses sacred knowledge in motion;
it hints at what it might mean to embody deep realization. This
dance, arising from the heart of space, is space's reply to the
unspoken question of our embodiment, the mystery of our being.
Here and now, space is dancing us.

KUM NYE DANCING FORMS

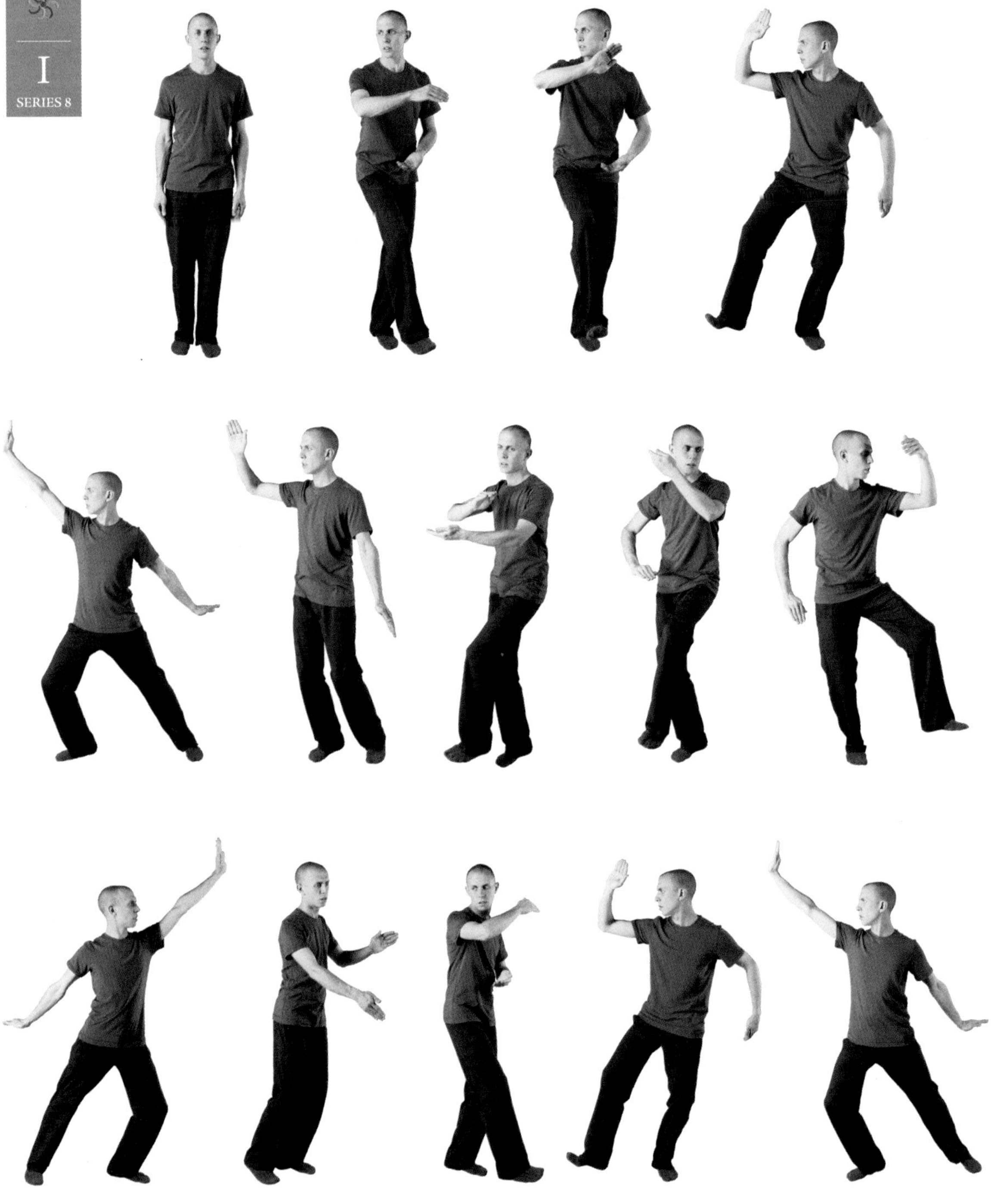

II

SERIES 8

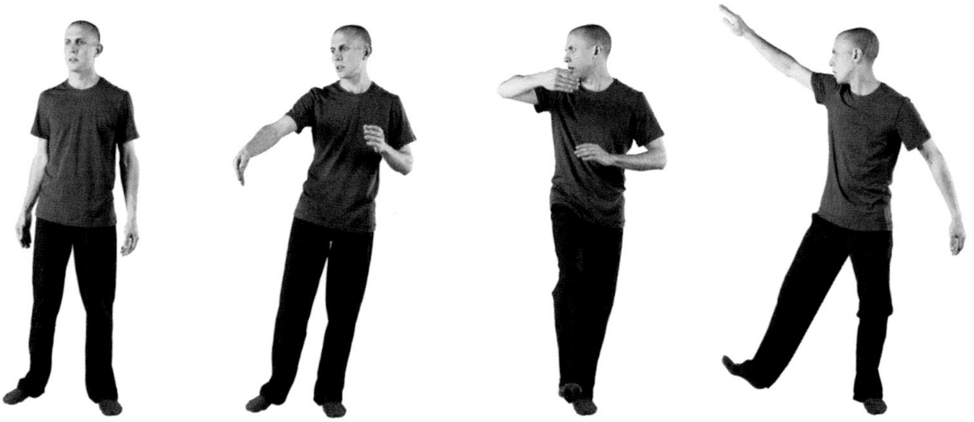

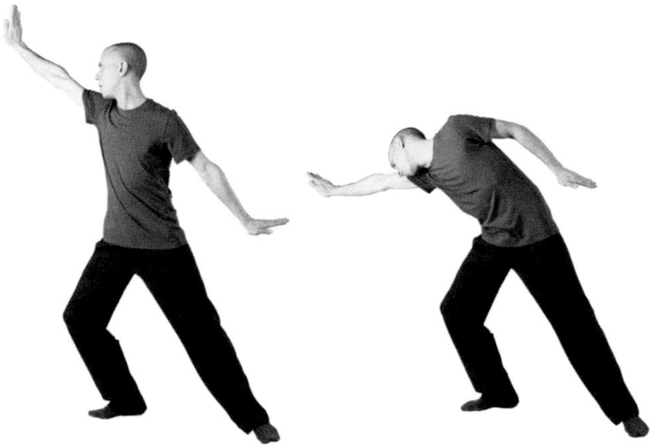

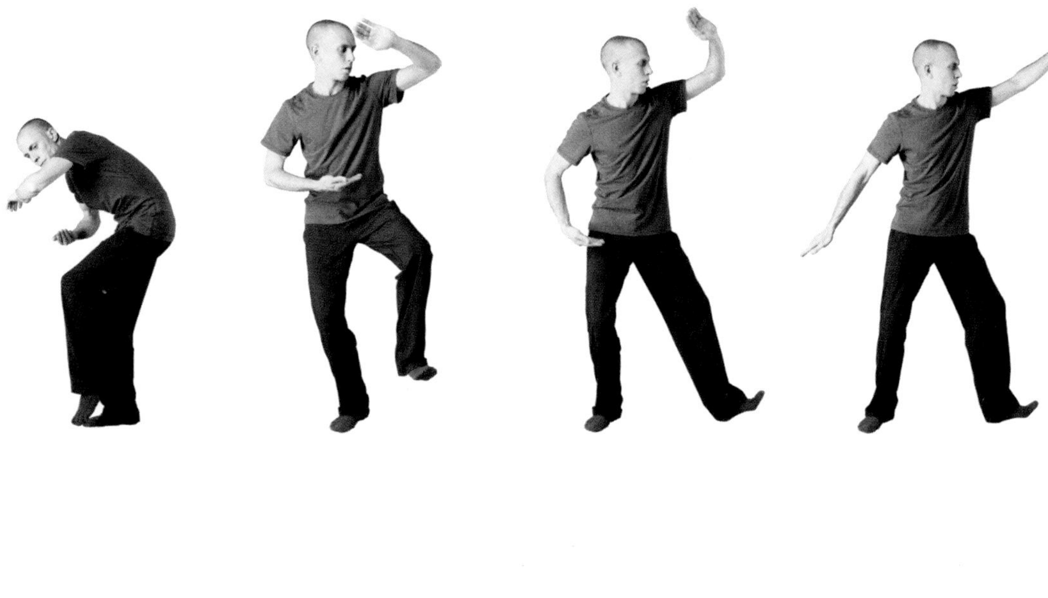

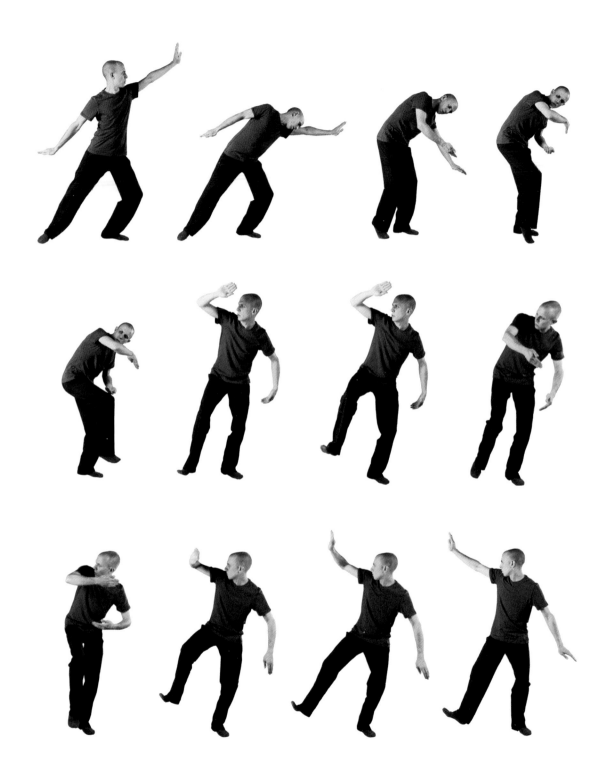

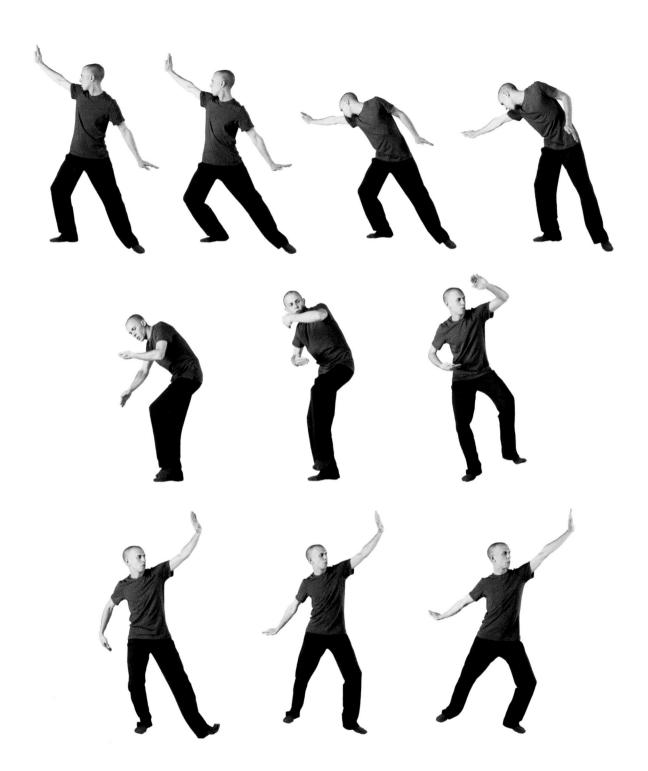

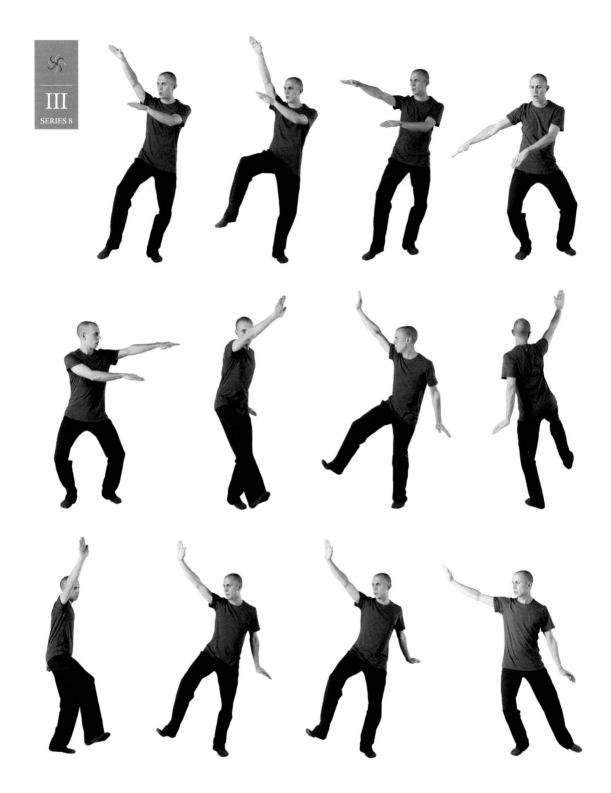

III
SERIES 8

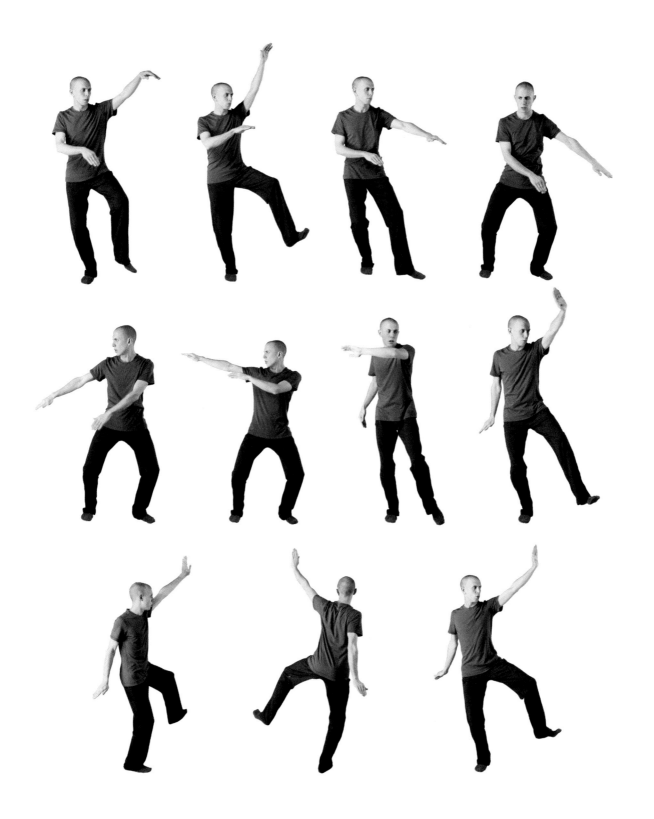

Index

Further learning can be done with an authorized teacher and through the Kum Nye Dancing DVDs (available through www.kumnyeyoga.com and www.dharmapublishing.com).

⋮

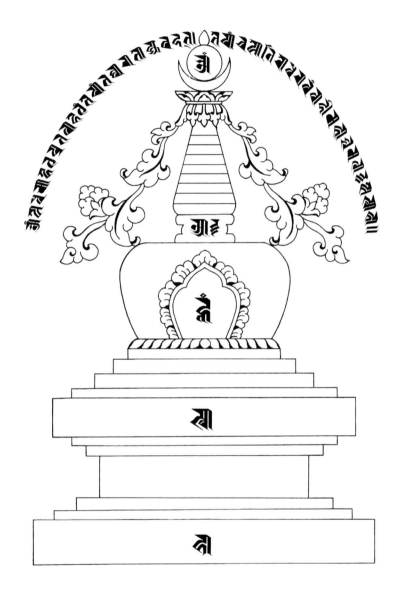